Beating Burnout

Physician Heal Thyself. A guide for busy, tired and stressed doctors.

By
Dr Phil Harley
MB BS (Lond), MRCGP, Blah Blah.

International copyright:
BrainSolutions 2016

All rights reserved.

ISBN-13: 978-1539508243

ISBN-10: 1539508242

"Stressed spelled backwards is desserts."

Anon.

Disclaimer

I do not know you or your life situation. This book is not intended to replace proper, prompt medical attention. So be a grown up and go and get some if you need some. This is intended to help you understand and recover from burnout. This contains sound medical advice in the abstract. But in the real world you have to take responsibility for yourself. Sorry about that.

Beating Burnout

Physician Heal Thyself. A guide for busy, tired and stressed doctors.

Introduction
1 Have I got burnout?
2 Just what exactly is burnout?
3 An official label
4 The slow burn
5 The causes
6 Increased pressure
7 The modern workplace
8 Twelve slippery steps
9 Burnout can make you sick
10 Why it matters
11 In a nutshell
12 A vocation
13 Move the goalposts
14 Locus of control
15 Pressures
16 Learn to say no
17 Journaling
18 Assumptions
19 Interpersonal conflict
20 We are pleasers
21 Being human
22 We cannot be seen to be weak
23 We cannot be ill
24 You are not a robot
25 The human physician
26 You are not a machine
27 Sleep

28 Downtime
29 Feeding
30 Being whelmed
31 Multi-tasking
32 Having a done list
33 Identity theft
34 Priorities
35 Are you depressed?
36 Do you become anxious?
37 Stress stuff
38 Self-care
39 Consultation antecedents
40 After seeing patients
41 Alcohol
42 Memory function
43 Drugs
44 Do you have Starbucks shares?
45 Smoking
46 What is your mental snooze alarm?
47 Procrastination
48 Workbook
49 Lifewheel
50 Goals
51 Healthy habits
52 Progressive relaxation
53 Mindfulness exercises
54 The end
55 About the author
56 References

introduction

Are you a tired physician? A busy doctor? A stressed parent?

Do you never have time to catch up? Do you ever get enough sleep? Do you have enough time to spend on you?

Are you getting on well with your family? Are you giving enough quality time to your partner? Do you keep your name badge on so your children can figure out who you are?

Do you need beer, gin or wine when you get home to unwind? Are you getting enough exercise (like what you tell your patients)? Do you have a great body shape, one which inspires your patients?

Are you crabby with colleagues? Do you get road rage? Do you sometimes shout at inanimate objects when they don't work properly or deliberately get in your way? Do other humans go out of their way to make your day more difficult? Does it feel like you are surrounded by idiots?

Do you get a lunch break? Do you leave a clear desk at work and finish your daily tasks with time to spare? Can you always focus well on the patient in front of you, giving your undivided attention, making them feel truly listened to? Do you have enough time for personal and professional development? Are you pressured by exams? Do you have to arrive early and leave late just to get somewhere close to managing the daily jobs?

Do your juniors find you easy going, approachable and supportive? Do you find enough time to teach in a learner centered way which you've pre-prepared (not a real word, I know) and read-up on? Are you able to keep up with the most important journals and the popular press articles which your patients may well bring as part of their ideas, concerns and expectations?

Do you make errors? If you notice them, do you pretend they didn't happen and hope no one else notices?

If reading this list resonates, giving a mildly depressive feeling of dread and recognition then you are not alone. You might be ok and it might all get better one day. But you may burn out. You may already be burned out or may be at significant risk of burning out.

Read on. You are among friends.

have I got burnout?

If the previous section sounded familiar, then the warning signs are there. Most authors agree that work pressures pile up causing stress (originally distress, only later becoming shortened). When the stress is prolonged, the person becomes detached and empty. This state is burnout.

If you notice that you aren't coping well all day every day, this is you at risk. A stress response is the normal reaction of an organism to environmental pressures and it is through this *hormesis* that we adapt and grow. But like all biological organisms, there is a finite level beyond which we don't thrive and the pressures become detrimental. It is this level of pressure or simply just the sustained relentless pressure that pushes us into no longer coping. This state of not coping is burnout. Like a spring sprung too far. Hook's law in humans. Like a perished elastic band. It is this we want to avoid. It takes a lot longer to correct and improve that stressed state once you've passed the point of easy spring back.

But stress is common in our profession. Perhaps nearly universal if we are honest enough.

I'm not saying you have poor coping strategies or are in some way weak if you feel pressure at work. But you are human and are likely to respond the way our brains do naturally to being under pressure.

I struggle. Not every day but some days. Currently I'm still working. I hope to keep it that way - it's a really handy way of paying the mortgage, the bills and paying for holidays for me and my family.

If I was independently really rich I'm not sure my day job is fulfilling enough to make me want to turn up at work. I may do, but it would be nice to have the choice about working. But this is the real world and I do have a mortgage.

I love my job (mostly). It's a great job, but seriously: The pressure is getting into silly proportions.

I'm a GP, (general practitioner, family physician, primary care doctor) in the UK. I think the stuff in this book applies pretty much across the board to all doctors. I will bring you the best of the evidence base and lead you through a few things that have really helped me, my patients and a good few of my colleagues.

This is a practical book and not one full of woo woo. Read it, hopefully not weep too much in recognition and go and try some of the practical pointers herein.

You are going to have to be creative if you are clutching the ebook. The printed version has margins to write in and I encourage you to make notes, scribbles and circles around what you find helpful (or even contest). The questions and exercises will work better if you actually do them. You can write all over the physical book if you are so minded. But a blank piece of paper from a nearby printer will do just fine.

I appreciate you're busy and pressured - otherwise you wouldn't be reading this. So the book and its chapters are short and pack a good powerful punch. A decent bang for your buck in terms of minutes involved for the results and measurable improvements in your QALYs.

Ok, I've not *actually* measured the QALYs but you get the idea. Grab some paper if you don't want to use a pen on the ereader, if you are using one.

Or buy the paperback and scribble all over it (this) in your favorite color wax crayon.

The British Medical Association suggest using the Oldenburg Burnout Inventory (OLBI) developed by Dr. Evangelia Demerouti (Demerouti and Bakker, 2008), which is felt to be a robust measurement tool (Reis, Xanthopoulou and Tsaousis, 2015). Burnout has been defined as *"an experience of physical, emotional, and mental exhaustion, caused by long-term involvement in situations that are emotionally demanding"*, with the prevalence in healthcare workers at nearly 25% (Mateen and Dorji, 2009).

Cole and Carlin (2009) stated: *"burnout is the index of dislocation between what people are and what they have to do. It represents an erosion in values, dignity, spirit, and will and erosion of the human soul"*. Although Descarte's assertion that the soul lived in the innocuous pineal gland didn't turn out to be correct (Russell, 1945), the sentiment is still valid even though the scientific detail inaccurate. The preservation of one's sense of soul seems to matter.

What exactly is burnout? Though the literature base is huge, it is a little fluffy and many authors try to put their own spin on what is essentially a word without form. The word means different things to different people at different times. However, common themes emerge. Most agree there are three main angles: **Physical exhaustion, emotional exhaustion and depersonalization.**

Physical and emotional exhaustion lead to low productivity. Worsening personal health follows. Often insidiously, physical symptoms mount. A decrease in mental wellbeing is the best barometer but difficult to notice in oneself and difficult to assess in another person, particularity one adept at showing a brave face and skilled at putting on a professional persona and facade to disguise one's true inner feelings. Having a profession which colludes with this approach is probably contributory. The teaching and guidance in one's early years, at least mine, was that you had to separate personal and professional. Not coping wasn't really an option. Not coping was weakness and not coping was seen to be largely your fault and it was up to you to sort it out.

This view is changing. But it is all too slow and the whole sea change required isn't forthcoming any time soon. Meanwhile we; our colleagues, you and I are threatened with approaching burnout. As we need help today, this week, this month or later this year, the drawn out five to ten year timescale of change or even longer is of no practical use to us.

Depersonalization is characterized by an internal feeling of low achievement (a mismatch between subjective and objective views), with a withdrawing from interpersonal interactions (patients, colleagues, family, friends). It feels like life is a daily trudge. This is different from the pressures of fast paced breathless work that is part of the response from stress - this is an extension of normal and relatively easily reversed. If persistent and not reversed, then burnout is the sequalae.

Burnout can occur in any occupation, though it occurs most often among the caring professions (Kakiashvili, Leszek and Rutkowski, 2013). It is the result of prolonged and cumulative emotional stress along with the pressures from interacting with the public on a daily basis.

just what exactly is burnout?

That's a good question and I'm glad you asked. You will of course have heard of it. But for most of us this is where the concrete knowledge ends. Again you are not alone. Experts disagree. There is no proper definition. Lots of people have their own definitions, but they vary. So I get to make one up too. Yay.

Burnout = *when the stress of the daily job grinds away for so long that all is left is an empty husk of your former magnificent self.*

Sounds bad doesn't it? It is. It is not without hope though. The sooner you spot it, the better. The sooner you recognize and acknowledge it for the reality that is biting, the sooner you are able to take steps to intervene.

That sounds a bit like the quasi-religiosity of the alcoholics anonymous' twelve steps. This book is not like that. It is about getting you better. It is about moving forwards in a carefully structured manner. It is about getting back in touch with who you used to be and building resilience, making you stronger for the future. There is nothing in these pages about higher powers and there are no affirmations. This is just practical, evidence based, smart advice from one doctor to another.

Physicians and doctors faced with stressful work without adequate recognition, reward and support are at risk of exhaustion (physical and emotional) and a developing detachment from their work. This accumulates and is frequently accompanied by decreased engagement, worsening concentration, increased frustration and emotional outbursts. Motivation wanes and the clinician no longer functions at their best.

Risk factors include:
- Younger doctors.
- Being a woman.
- Perceived high workload.
- Perceived inadequate resources.
- Poor support (colleagues and family).
- A poor understanding of where you fit into the machine.

Stress is different to burnout. Some define stress as being too much pressure, here people feel that if they can just work a bit harder or that if some magical event were to occur, then everything would be ok again. This is good. It shows there is still hope (however unrealistic) and this engenders a mindset to accompany it. This set of circumstances could also do with being changed for long term health and wellbeing, but the crisis isn't yet upon us.

Burnout is a set of negative emotions. Being empty, uncaring, devoid of hope with all the optimism dried up. You will notice stress but burnout can creep up insidiously.

Stress has a sense of urgency and deadlines. Type A personality and behaviors. Engaged but barely coping with the hamster wheel. You may die from a hypertensive heart-attack or stroke. Burnout differs, it culminates in a depersonalized husk of the former self. Not even noticing or caring if there is a wheel. Hopeless and helpless to act, lacking in energy for anything. Depressive and ahedonic and much more at risk of death from a completed suicide.

an official label

Burnout is an official ICD-10 diagnosis: a life management disorder (ICD-10, 2015).

Labeling is a bit of a double edged sword.

It's great that the term is recognized in that this opens doors to access helpful stuff; occupational health support and official validation. It can be less helpful in that it also opens the doors for wallowing in a sick-role, which can hinder speedy recovery. There is also the pesky problem of actually admitting it is becoming a problem and allowing the facade of being an invulnerable immortal to slip. It's not just you and I. That doesn't come very easily for any physician and the cultural assumptions we adhere to perpetuate this unhelpful social construct. More on this later.

Burnout is an extreme of a perfectly normal phenomenon; which is feeling pretty rough when the pressures mount up. And at some point you break and become less functional or even non-functioning.

It is to identify and prevent this, then to recover from it - that this guide you have eagerly clutched in your paws is about.

You do it for other people; you care about them, you help them. Why not do this for you? It is time to look after yourself. Turn your brain, skills and life experience onto someone who matters. Someone who counts. You. Do it for you, for your family, for your friends, for the patients you meet each day and those you have yet to help.

ICD10 states burnout symptoms = **physical and mental**

exhaustion on minimal effort.
- *Myalgia.*
- *Dizziness.*
- *Tension type headaches.*
- *Poor sleep.*
- *Inability to relax.*
- *Irritability.*
- *Inability to recover after rest, relaxation or entertainment...*

Which sounds a lot like the biological symptoms of depression and generalized anxiety disorder rolled into one. They last for more than three months and aren't explained by other illnesses.

Stress responses are normal, they are actually good. They evolved to keep us safe. Like running away from saber toothed tigers. The problem comes when the stressor - having a tiger nearby, lasts for a long time.

In our evolutionary past the acute pressures didn't usually last very long. We got eaten or ran away. Now we can become chronically stressed about an impending tax bill, working in a department run by morons or a daily clinic full of heartsinks; these stresses and pressures can last for hours, days and even weeks or months.

Our bodies and brains simply don't do very well when exposed to the constant hyper-arousal state this produces. It may be excess cortisol, it may be heightened sensitivity to circulating catecholamines, which themselves may be elevated above baseline. It could be insulin, it may be raised IL-1 or suppressed IL-GF. We don't really know for sure. It could be a little bit of everything.

What we do know is that to do well, to live, thrive and survive we need adequate decent quality downtime. We need to feel valued. We need to be pushed, tested and intellectually and emotionally engaged in meaningful work. BUT in a supportive environment which is heavy on the rewards. The paid rewards don't seem to matter nearly as much as praise and recognition or the occasionally unexpected bonus reward; though perhaps counterintuitive, it is evidence based (Lepper et al, 1973; Baranek, 1996; Peyton, 1998; Jaremko and Meichenbaum, 2013).

If we don't have engaging work with adequate support and recognition - we feel worse each day and everything starts to go a bit awry. It typically sinks in a slowly downward spiral until the situation is reversed by paying attention to self-care, setting boundaries and asking for help.

What is Burnout?
> *"A state of physical, emotional, and mental exhaustion caused by long term involvement in emotionally demanding situations."*
> (Malach-Pines and Giora, 2005)

"A state of fatigue or frustration brought about by devotion to a cause, way of life, or relationship that failed to produce the expected reward."
(Freudenberger and Richelson, 1980)

It is when you are:
- Emotionally exhausted.
- Mentally exhausted.
- Depersonalized (that burnt out husk feeling).

The cause is stress (lots of it over a long time). You feel this stress when you cannot cope with demands. You feel overwhelmed and that the demands are unrelenting. You start to lose sight of your original motivators. Of why you wanted to be a doctor in the first place.

Your energy goes down, your productivity follows. You are left feeling helpless and powerless to change you or the situation. You become resentful, increasingly cynical and when you have nothing left to give, you are left as an empty husk. A burned out shell of your former self. It is this negativity that characterizes burnout over stress.

Stress is simply pressure. We all have pressured days and weeks. When this is unrelenting and our recharge capacity is not keeping pace for whatever reason; this is when the slide towards burnout occurs. Becoming bored at work isn't nice but is not as risky as being perpetually overloaded while feeling unappreciated. Keeping all the plates spinning requires us to be functioning at full capacity. Anything that nibbles away at our coping strategies and our sense of identity will eventually burn us out. There are personal predisposing factors sure, but eventually probably all of us will burnout if given the right, or should I say the wrong circumstances.

It is not a sign of weakness or lack of character in the same way the truly depressed patient is a victim of his or her personal neurochemistry at that point. We wouldn't blame them any more than we blame an epileptic for having a seizure. Similarly burnout is the the outward manifestation of a whole set of circumstances that have conspired to take a physician out of useful circulation.

We can all become exhausted. Burnout happens with repeated exhaustion plus ongoing stress while being undermined. Undermined by having insufficient supporting measures in place. A table without enough working table legs. Internal supports *(mental wellbeing, adequate sleep, rest and downtime, good physical health)* and external supports *(adequate resources, praise and recognition, autonomy and a sense of purpose and meaning grounded in values which are aligned to your own value system)*.

The feckless and lazy become exhausted and unmotivated. That's not you or me. We are are risk of burnout - this is worse. It takes longer to put right and isn't sorted out in a weekend. Working harder doesn't make burnout go away. It makes it worse. Burnout strikes at those who are, or at least have been highly committed. It is said you can only burn out if you've been properly alight to begin with.

We all have off days. Days when staying under the duvet and not emerging seems to be the best plan. Days when we are juggling too many balls and people are kicking us in the shins and shouting in our ears. Days when simply everything that can go wrong does. That's ok. Not nice, but ok; simply a part of life. But when that feels like a normal day and you dread going to work because it is always horrible, unrewarding and you find yourself shouting at inanimate objects like the toaster, that isn't so good. Days when you snap at people and wish they would stop bothering you and simply leave you alone. These are clues you may be burning out.

Big fat hairy clues:
- Every day is a bad day.
- Putting efforts into your work or home life seems pointless.
- You're perpetually exhausted.
- Most of your day is spent fire-fighting.
- Nihilism rules. You strongly feel nothing you do will make a difference anyway. Yet with cognitive dissonance you still manage to worry and stress over what you do or say.

What to do:
- **Spot it**: Look for and heed the warning signs.
- **Stop:** Take a big breath and stop the deluge of pressure. Move the goal posts. Take time out. Ask for help.
- **Start over:** Realign your priorities. Reassess your goals. Look for a silver lining. Work on your locus of control.
- **Be future proof:** Win the lottery and move to the Bahamas. Actually, I mean put in place stuff which will hopefully avoid this happening again. Keep vigilant. Look after yourself (body, mind and spirit). Buy my other books (maybe ;) Eat better, sleep more, exercise more. Do fun stuff. Set inspirational and aspirational motivating goals. Connect with loved ones. Do random acts of kindness. Be kind to your patients and small furry animals and so on. Work on your resilience to stress by taking better care of your physical and emotional health. Then teach others to do likewise.

Do any of these feel familiar?
- Dreading the work day before it has begun.
- Clock watching, wishing the day was over.
- Lack of interest at work.
- Having no functional capacity to get dressed properly, let alone cope with what your patients have in store for you.
- Feeling that you can't deal with your own life, so how can you help any patients deal with theirs?

- Insomnia. Feeling inadequately rested when you are woken by your alarm.
- Not being able to remember the last time you slept in, woken by the sun and took a leisurely breakfast.
- Not being able to remember that last time you took a properly relaxing holiday.
- Finding excuses not to go to work. Leaving late, arriving late.
- Are you checking job adverts to see if there is a better role available?
- Are you wanting to go part time, take early retirement or throw in the towel, feeling an urge to go and open a beach front bar or coffee shop?
- Do you feel emotionally drained and empty?
- Do you have a permanently sore throat, a mild cough and muscle aches? Is your posture terrible and are your frown wrinkles deepening by the day?
- Are you experiencing physical complaints such as headaches, illness, or backache?
- Do you want to shout at people, even though deep down you know it isn't their fault (for being stupid and getting in your way)?
- Having thoughts that your work doesn't have meaning or make a difference.
- Are you unappreciated at work and at home?
- Are you disconnecting from your family and friends because you simply don't have the spare emotional capacity, time or energy to maintain these relationships? Do you look for excuses to drop out of or decline social engagements, often at the last minute? Having attacks of the 'fake gastric flu syndrome' or migraines.

the slow burn

Burnout is not new. It is a word for something real but ephemeral. It is a concept. You cannot touch it, you cannot put some in a wheelbarrow. Its roots are from a novel by Graham Green (A Burnt-Out Case) who's protagonist is suffering burnout. Inspired by this, psychologist Herbert Freudenberger published on medical staff burnout in the 1970's. Gradually it became understood to mean a state of exhaustion, poor motivation and impaired effectiveness (Freudenberger, 1974).

Occupational burnout is frequently found in professions who are front facing to the public. The two common components are a high stress environment and an emotionally demanding role. Doctors are therefore front and center when it comes to risk.

The diagnosis of burnout is included in the ICD-10 under the heading 'Other specified nonpsychotic mental disorders'. The features quoted are:
> *"A mental disorder characterized by chronic fatigue and concomitant physiologic symptoms. It cites psychogenic fatigue as an approximate synonym."*

How can you tell if you have it? There are many questionnaires you can complete. These have the merit of being quick and easy, but have inherent problems of validity and reproducibility. Even then the definitions of burnout itself vary. The Maslach Burnout Inventory is one of the more widely used scales of attempting to quantify burnout (Maslach, Jackson and Leiter, 1996). The three components are exhaustion, cynicism, and inefficacy. Others have argued that just exhaustion is needed to diagnose burnout (Shirom and Melamed, 2005).

You could say that the precise definition doesn't matter. If you are stressed to the point you are ill and no longer effective you probably have it. If you are not coping well and are becoming ill, you are probably either developing it or are at serious risk. The point here is that there is help and this is more effective if sought early. Burnout is a thing, a real thing and left unchecked has dire, unpleasant and sad consequences for us physicians (Bianchi et al, 2015).

Burnout shares a lot of similar symptoms with depression. There is certainly a degree of overlap and there may indeed be a spectrum. The two can co-exist and may be addressed together or separately. But the semantics perhaps don't matter. The treatments are similar and the approaches to moving forward overlap too. Where we should draw the diagnostic wording is currently not clear and it is also not clear if this distinction is worthy of more research.

Some people will be more accepting of burnout as a diagnosis and some of depression. This will have to do with their life experiences and working knowledge of both.

I would argue the distinction is immaterial from an approach perspective, but could be very important for the patient. Some doctors approaching burnout may find it less stigmatizing than a diagnosis of depressive illness and some *vice versa* (Andrew, 2006 and Miles, 1998). As long as there is minimal stigma and the diagnosis allows each patient to move forward fastest and most effectively while enabling them to ask for and receive appropriate support in their personal and professional life, then whichever diagnosis fits better - use that one.

increased pressure

The information revolution allows more and more data to be processed ever more effectively and our social and job roles are evolving rapidly to try and keep pace.

The drive for ever greater efficiencies and profits accelerates year on year. Patient expectations rise annually. The politicians promise ever greater things for ever lower taxes and rashly promise increases in healthcare spending while slashing budgets. In the background medical knowledge continues apace in every single specialty. We can do ever more for our patients and they expect ever more, while becoming less mentally adept at understanding the cost-benefits of their expensive treatments and are less tolerant of medical paternalisim. They are increasingly quick to litigate over things they should have perhaps thought through properly before pressuring their physician in the first place. The whole of medicine and medical knowledge is growing exponentially but much of this research is funded by pharmaceutical giants with studies performed against placebo rather than against the previous gold-standard widely available and cheaper treatment. The studies are skewed and biased with missing data on exclusions and minimal proven benefits but massive advertising budgets. These emotive drivers push our patients to demand of us what is not always in their best interests and as a profession we are ever more accountable in ever more unreasonable circumstances.

It is no wonder that some people find the day job increasingly challenging.

We have to be permanently polite and empathic, be ever more patient centered and are held to be permanently accountable for everything we do or say to patients, their relatives, our staff, the press, the public and even in our own personal lives.

So while there isn't the published evidence that burnout is mounting in every specialty. I think we don't need these studies. Be real, be practical. We are pretty much all at risk. We should remain vigilant. And if you have better coping strategies than me, you can probably think of a colleague who may be at risk or need some help.

NHS England in April 2016 stepped up its £3.5million project by another sixteen million to provide a dedicated occupational health service to their general practitioners. The previous chair of the Royal College of General Practitioners said she could often not distinguish between doctors and patients with post traumatic stress disorder. Dr Phil Hammond stated:

> *"It's deeply ironic and paradoxical that we are harming and possibly killing, the very people looking after us. We need to address that."*

Post-traumatic stress disorder is defined in ICD-10 as:
- *A class of traumatic stress disorders with symptoms that last more than one month.*
- There are various forms of post-traumatic stress disorder, depending on the time of onset and the duration of these stress symptoms. In the acute form, the duration of the symptoms is between 1 to 3 months. In the chronic form, symptoms last more than 3 months. With delayed onset, symptoms develop more than 6 months after the traumatic event.
- Acute, chronic, or delayed reactions to traumatic events such as military combat, assault, or natural disaster.
- An anxiety disorder precipitated by an experience of intense fear or horror while exposed to a traumatic (especially life-threatening) event. The disorder is characterized by intrusive recurring thoughts or images of the traumatic event; avoidance of anything associated with the event; a state of hyperarousal and diminished emotional responsiveness. These symptoms are present for at least one month and the disorder is usually long-term.
- An anxiety disorder that develops in reaction to physical injury or severe mental or emotional distress, such as military combat,

violent assault, natural disaster, or other life-threatening events. Having cancer may also lead to post-traumatic stress disorder. Symptoms interfere with day-to-day living and include reliving the event in nightmares or flashbacks; avoiding people, places, and things connected to the event; feeling alone and losing interest in daily activities; and having trouble concentrating and sleeping (ICD-10, 2015).

Post-traumatic stress disorder (PTSD) is a real illness. You can get PTSD after living through or seeing a traumatic event. PTSD makes you feel stressed and afraid after the danger is over. It affects your life and the people around you. PTSD can cause problems like:
- *flashbacks, or feeling like the event is happening again.*
- *trouble sleeping or nightmares.*
- *feeling alone.*
- *angry outbursts.*
- *feeling worried, guilty or sad.*

It doesn't seem too much of a stretch to agree that burnout shares many of these characteristics.

PTSD starts at different times for different people. Signs of PTSD may start soon after a frightening event and then continue. Other people develop new or more severe signs months or even years later. PTSD can happen to anyone, even children. Medicines can help you feel less afraid and tense. It might take a few weeks for them to work. Talking to a specially trained doctor or counselor also helps many people with PTSD. This (amazingly) is called talk therapy. Talking therapies are often effective in physicians as they are articulate, with the solution oriented behavioral and cognitive approaches tapping into their dispassionate skills.

This PTSD response may result from a focal point of stress such as a complaint, case which went wrong, or being called before your medical board.

Again, not really a surprise that some doctors cope, some do not cope, but a great many squirrel away their emotions with this emerging later as burnout or post-traumatic stress disorder.

The approaches to cure are the same; so again do not get caught up too much in the semantics. If the semantics will change the stigma, the help available and not engender a sick-role (the only thing wrong with that is that progress tends to be poor), then pick whichever diagnostic label fits better and tailor treatment from there (Kraft, 2006).

Doctors are a specific subset of the population, as they have all the same pressures as the general workforce but are forced through social and professional conventions to be a swan and to never admit fallibility or any type of personal vulnerability, lest the thin veneer of super-human god-like capacity fall away or be stripped down.

Many cling to this as a coping mechanism and medical school encourages it. The junior doctor intern years bolster this and ingrain unhealthy coping strategies. In the next ten years everything else falls apart, you become functionally dysfunctional or come to be an exception and somehow survive by luck and good genes, aided by a supportive background.

Burnout is a bit like stress fractures:
- due to repeated stress.
- due to a *straw that broke the camel's back* moment.
- worse with underlying predispositions.
- better with rest.
- do recover.
- recover with predictable patterns.
- can still function with one but suboptimal and not going to help healing.
- they hurt.
- you can get another (in the same or a different place).
- they should ring alarm bells about the workload of what you are doing each day. Are you simply asking too much?
- a reminder that despite what you do being fabulous and groovy and despite all appearances to the contrary (either in your head or in the real world), you are NOT super-human ... sorry about that.

Stress is unfortunate, becoming burned out is awful. While identifying this is important, *do* just check you aren't in actual fact ill:

- Unexplained weight loss (if you're not sure, then do weekly weights).
- Bone pain.
- Night pains.
- Persistent change in bowel habit (irritable bowel syndrome will fluctuate, cancer tends to stick to one pattern and stay there).
- Stress can cause reflux, but won't make your stools darker.
- Low back pain can be multiple myeloma but won't improve with keeping active with better posture as the mechanical causes will.
- Neck pains from stress improve with a massage. Other ones don't tend to.
- Stress headaches don't usually cause vomiting or any signs of raised intracranial pressure / field defects or focal neurological deficit.
- Thyroid disorders, low vitamin D, anaemia and leukaemias are relatively common causes of feeling dreadful and can be readily detected by blood tests from your own family physician.

the causes

Burnout has many causes. This multifactoral etiology is then predisposed to by personal factors. This makes sense. Life circumstances and personality produce much of the variance in our patients, with some populations being more at risk of being affected than others. And within susceptible populations; life events, gene expression, personality traits and life skills such as resilience also play a role. This is not new or controversial.

People become burned out when their stress coping mechanisms are overwhelmed. The causes will vary on each occasion and with each person. The trouble with burnout is that the onset is insidious and the consequences dire (Ruotsalainen et al, 2014).

Early recognition and early intervention would seem manifestly important, though there is currently no evidence in the literature to confirm or refute this. Designing studies to research this would be expensive and are unlikely to have the power needed to draw firm conclusions. So, just like so much in medicine and in real life, we will have to make an educated guess about how best to address this challenge on a day to day basis in the unscientific and complex cauldron that is the real life we get up to each day and immerse ourselves in.

Work factors impact on burnout. Rising expectations, decreasing resources and increased accountability all take their toll.

Expectations are soaring of the medical profession. Above and beyond the working week. This is the difference between a job and a profession, but is it normal to respond to emails / tweets / texts at all hours of day and night?

Are we addicted to the rush of the info? The urgency of a ringing phone can transfer to every electronic communication. And they are never off. Should they be?

Accessing work stuff online from home is the thin end of a wedge, a slippery slope akin to campaign drift or mission creep seen in combat theaters. Checking blood results, writing letters or referrals, going through complaints. Because some of it is expected of us, we are thought of badly if we do not toe the line.

Some of us have boundaries and won't work in the evenings once we are home. So much so that one GP partner I know was fired as her colleagues deemed her acopic - they could see she was processing blood reports at ten in the evening from home. They assumed rather than being diligent, that she wasn't competent enough to handle to working day and fired her ass. She may actually have been appropriately partitioning and crow barring in lots of down-time during the working day and was functioning well, all at harmony in her body, mind and spirit.

I don't know and wasn't there. But it highlights the fine line to be trod. The challenge is that we are social creatures and judge others and hold them to standards that we ourselves rarely meet. Somebody else's lines and definitions will differ from ours, but we all keep them to ourselves in our own heads without generally sharing them. Then we have the temerity to think ill of those who don't match our (invisible and varying) impossibly high standards.

What exactly is work-life balance? Is it all work? Is it work at the expense of life or the other way around? Why can you only have one or the other at any one time? It is such an easy phrase to say and because it has passed into popular use, few of us stop to consider what it really means. It is usually thought to talk about making sure you have enough life outside work to maintain your sanity and dare I say get some enjoyment out of life.

We are accountable. All day every day. As doctors we hold a place in society that affords us certain privileges. We are allowed to help people, we are mostly exempt from assault charges (examining people is common assault, but we usually act as if we have implied consent). We command a reasonably high wage and a lot of people hold the members of our profession in high esteem.

The flip side is that we are expected always to behave in a manner commensurate with that role. We should behave with decorum at all times in work and out. We are expected to behave as if we are representing the reputations of the entire profession. You could argue the rights and wrongs of this, but it is the case. Many professional board cases relate to behavior relating to these standards.

We are also highly accountable at work for everything we do, write and say. All of these can be held against us by anybody for decades. This can feel pretty stressful. No unguarded comments can ever be said or written, either in the consultation or in the corridor.

This permanent accountability is becoming ever more intense as the public feel they should exert greater control over doctors' decision making and thus their professional lives. The popular press ever more delights in the transgressions of physicians. Online records and permanent electronic recordings of voice calls and patients videoing consultations on their phones means that this is burgeoning. The public is also ever keener to litigate and press charges. Either in the pursuit of an easy buck or as a personal self-righteous crusade when they perceive their inalienable rights have been breached.

The short version is that this can be stress inducing, is getting worse by the day and will continue to do so for your entire career. It may be time now to make some peace with that situation as you aren't going to stem that particular tide by sulking.

But what can we do? We could try and regain some of our lost power. If you have power you feel good. If you don't feel you have power that feels bad. So the more autonomy you perceive you have the better. It doesn't have to be real, It has only to seem real. But your workload is often outside your control and you may have to work to externally imposed contracts.

Managing the stressors in each of our lives is an ongoing challenge that we need to keep a careful eye on. Stressors such as complaints and litigation are ever increasing and making us ill (Charles and Frisch, 2005; Balch et al, 2011; Bourne et al, 2015). We need to act to save our health, with early intervention being easier, like correcting the course of a ship. Small rudder movements are the key to effective yacht racing. Tiny adjustments to keep you on course. To keep track of something insidious, sometimes it is enough to simply consider it in a dispassionate manner periodically and trying to keep it not too far from the front of your mind. Assessment at our annual appraisal may be sufficient for some of us. Using the validated tools can help. But this light touch approach comes at a risk: **You might not spot burnout approaching.**

I feel that this is a complex area and the tools are simply just tools. The best scoring system available is no doubt excellent, but at best dim candlelight to guide our way. They are, however an excellent starting point, a useful way to engage with the process and a handy method for opening up a dialog with mentors, colleagues, or our own physician if we take this complex problem to them. Stay alert to burnout. Don't over-diagnose it, certainly. But the risks of missing it are not insignificant either (Cole and Carlin, 2009).

It would seem that burnout is becoming more prevalent (Alarcon, Eschleman and Bowling, 2009). Again, sadly there is no conclusive evidence but data from the Mayo clinic supports this (Shanafelt et al 2015). It could be that it is becoming accepted and part of the zeitgeist, in that more people are aware of it. It may be becoming less stigmatized, allowing more people to come out of the closet and openly discuss their burnout. It could be a genuine increase in prevalence. It may be a shift of labeling from the alternative and often overlapping diagnoses of depression and the rather woolly terms; stress and mental breakdown. It may be a more medicalized and thus acceptable moniker, attracting more help than simply labeling it as stress. The split for me being that stress is a temporary thing, easily reversed and burnout is what happens when lots of stressed days mount up without adequate respite (with ensuing gradual depersonalization). Burnout is the result from a chronic accumulation of stress (rather than an acute mismatch in pressures and resources available to manage them).

I'm also alarmed to note that among us family physicians the numbers are not only soaring but approaching silly proportions. In family medicine 51.3 percent of physicians reported burnout in 2011 versus 63.0 percent in 2014. A twenty per cent climb over three years. And these numbers are two years behind the curve with the inevitable delays with proper publication (Shanafelt et al, 2015).

the modern workplace

Burnout is claimed to be increasing because of the evolving modern workplace. I'm not sure this is true (Dale and Olds, 2012). The workplace is changing and burnout is increasing but no causal conclusions can be drawn from two axiomatic statements. That is sloppy science. Variables aren't necessarily dependent and even when they are, the relationship could be directly linear, inversely related, or more complex. Life is complex. Many interdependent variables abound. Work environments have always wanted more for less from their employees. There have always been a range of coping capacities within the workforce to soak up the pressures. This inbuilt and home grown resilience varies between individuals and even within individuals. It may be that there is a parallel to be drawn with public expectations of people in a certain role and how these are changing in one particular direction. All speeded up with the rate of change of societal norms which have been revolutionized over the last two decades by the explosion of information technology (Cole and Carlin, 2009).

The pressure on young people, real or imagined to conform to societal norms such as beauty and body shape seems ever more pervasive. The perfect smile, the blemish-less face, the unrealistic athletic, toned body radiating sex appeal in a persona comfortable in crowds, self-confident, intellectually robust and financially successful seems to be the ideal we hold ourselves to. We strive to live the playboy, celebrity lifestyle but with finite resources, our own less fortunate genetics and very real budget constraints. We also have real life intruding with ailing relatives, tax bills to meet, the school-run to do and limited capacity for the spare time to even manage to munch some lunch during what other people call the working day. We are expected to be the perfect spouse, to never grump or grouse, to be charming to all we meet and to be great conversation at a dinner party, which incidentally we should have prepared after the working day and should resemble something from a Michelin starred restaurant. And did I mention the beach-ready body that somehow I seem to be missing?

These social pressures seem to be on the increase while the pressures on qualified doctors moves in the same direction (Freudenberger and Géraldine, 1980; Andrew, 2006). Some of the pressures represent a real raising of standards and may be worth pursuing. But some or many may be less reasonable or realistic. Some of these pressures only actually exist in our own heads as assumptions and we don't perhaps need to be questing in the wake of unrealistic role-models who aren't actually so perfect in the real world.

If we aren't careful we can find ourselves chasing some unachievable ideal, some picture of perfection and hold ourselves up against this. When we inevitably come up short, we then start an unhelpful internal dialog which berates us for not being good enough, for not trying enough and although this is meant to be a mental pep-talk to spur our efforts ever skywards, can end up becoming a self-defeating negative influence on our daily moods.

Stress can be viewed as the **mismatch between job demands and job resources**, with burnout as the non-functioning burned out self that awaits the chronically stressed. These demands are both physical and psychological. Time pressures, exertional demands and logistical challenges along with pressure from above and the public (real or perceived) together with mental processing, decision making and emotional trauma. Job resources are things that help workers meet these demands. But who has enough of these? Demerouti et al (2001) claim exhaustion is correlated to job demands and that disengagement is negatively correlated with job resources; saying exhaustion comes with demands and workers disengage if resources are inadequate. Not really a surprise.

Maslach, Schaufeli and Leiter (2001) gave us six risk factors for

burnout:
- mismatch in workload.
- mismatch in control.
- lack of appropriate awards.
- loss of a sense of positive connection with others in the workplace.
- perceived lack of fairness.
- conflict between values.

Some academics view burnout as a sequence. This sequence could be thought of like the stages of grieving / receiving bad news. **Denial, anger, bargaining, depression and acceptance** (Kübler-Ross, 1969).

All stages may well be present. Most of the time. Though not for everyone. Not necessarily in the same order and stages can overlap (Kraft, 2006). Meaning that although a useful set of hooks to start hanging ideas and linking experience to: This is just a list of things that you may find useful. Don't set too much stock in it - but it is a good place to start if you need some launch point to springboard your journey, or common ground to explore in conversations with patients, colleagues or mentors.

As a physician you are at risk of burnout from your **personal qualities**. I've not met you, but you are likely to be conscientious, hard-working, highly motivated and committed. You are probably compassionate, have high ideals and are willing to sacrifice some of yourself in order to help others. This helping is tied to our identities - and can be untied, but only if we come to understand better the 'who' it happens to in the first place - and there *are* ways to untie without losing personal and professional face.

If we are able to deliberately disconnect our sense of self and our professional persona, this could bring more productivity and better personal resilience. This is a vital part of ongoing professional development (Mateen and Dorji, 2009).

Type A personalities are more prone to stress and its sequalae. This was quite revolutionary in its day - but we've moved on and have learned to recognize the world as a bit (a lot) more complex than that. Medicine is full of perfectionists, unable to relax unless everything is done just right. This is characterized by not delegating effectively. While this is not inherently bad if things are going well, if they are not: address this. Now.

Physicians have a tendency to be competitive work-driven controllers. We fight against deadlines and want to dominate. This shouldering of the workload is not sustainable, errors creep in. But due to the facade and image (real / imagined / internal and external) we feel we need to maintain - we sometimes cope less well when the errors are spotted / happen and are noticed / have an impact.

Then we deny / hide / cover up / make excuses / blame others. Like a cornered wild animal we can lash out - physically / orally / emotionally against anyone (sometimes the easy prey - like loved ones at home). Or we hide and deny (ostrich style). Ostriching can result in unhealthy coping behavior (drugs / affairs / overwork - taking on even more stuff just to prove you are still coping).

Sometimes ostrich behavior can appear constructive: More courses, qualifications / conferences / more academia. But this all too often proves to no avail. This is a veneer. Of no substance, it is just *papering over the cracks*. We need to retain a sense that we too are human. This isn't just useful and helpful but is vital. Especially if we are to maintain any sense of vitality or achieve longevity.

The external forces that affect our daily work lives will only go up. We don't live in a world where stuff suddenly gets easier and although I'm an optimist, I'm not stupid. In the modern workplace many of us become stressed, while not everyone burns out. So what is the difference? The difference between simple stress and burnout isn't crystal clear. There is no precise dividing line. The accepted wisdom is that **stress is a normal reaction**. A physical and mental response to pressures. If you work harder or have the pressures magically removed, then you will feel better after a weekend, or a week long vacation.

Burnout on the other hand is the long term thing. That state of physical and emotional exhaustion and emptiness that has a real disconnect, with true disengagement at its heart.

That all sounds pretty bad. Do we know what causes burnout? Not really. There is no one single cause of burnout. Many factors contribute. Personal and professional factors both count. The more there are stacking up, the more likely burnout is to follow. Lack of autonomy is a leading contributor. Lack of meaning in your work is cited in the journals as a leading cause of burnout. In medicine, most of us start from a place of finding the work very meaningful and most applicants to medical school cite it as their leading driver for applying.

As the years go by and the dew lifts from our idealistic twenty-something eyes, we see the world more for how it really is and a certain sense of cynicism can develop. This can be a coping strategy to handle the myriad emotional challenges of practising medicine. But it can also be a sign of burnout developing. An increasing sense of pointlessness about one's job role is a warning sign.

Is the nihilism biting? We are all going to die anyway, so are all of my patients, if I stop them dying today they will simply die of something else another day. These thoughts and feelings are to some extent natural and normal extrapolations of logical processes that any inquiring and intelligent mind capable of lateral and logical thought may entertain from time to time. But if this nihilism pervades your working day and affects your patient interactions, then this should be considered. And in depth.

It's certainly not my view that you should disregard intellectual questioning of the role of the physician. Quite the opposite. But if your internal machinations and the rights, wrongs and wherewithals of your job role impact on your patient interactions, then these should all be considered carefully. Anything that negatively impacts on patients should be considered for review and removal from your mental scripts. This is central to modern reflective practise.

If you feel that you may be burning or burned out, action is needed. If you feel permanently stressed and dread going to work, finding excuses to call in sick, you should view this as highly suspicious that burnout is a risk if not actually having already arrived.

twelve slippery steps down

Is this you? Burnout steps can be thought of sequentially as:

1 - Compulsion to prove oneself
It can start as excessive ambition. The desire to prove oneself becomes compulsion.

2 - Working harder
To prove themselves to others or fit in, people set high personal expectations. To meet these they focus solely on work while taking on more work than they should. They do everything themselves to try and prove themselves irreplaceable.

3 - Neglecting their needs
Everything revolves around work with no time and energy for anything else. Like friends and family, eating and sleeping are relegated to secondary importance.

4 - Displacement of conflicts
They develop awareness that something is wrong, but cannot see that work and their approach is the source of this issue. This can feel like a personal crisis and biological features appear.

5 - Revision of values
Value systems change. Work becomes the new norm. This consumes all available physical and emotional resources; leaving none for family, social life or hobbies. People become emotionally blunted.

6 - Denial of emerging problems
People may withdraw when their capacity to engage socially becomes diminished, as physical and emotional resources are channeled into work activities. They may come across as

behaving in a socially inappropriate manner or become defensive or even aggressive. Particularly if this behavior is questioned, pointed out or challenged. They are likely to deny the problem is within themselves and attribute any actions or behavior to an external locus of control and explain everything in terms of pressure put upon them from outside and the lack of available resources to match these, despite their manifestly obvious (to them) efforts and achievements to keep things on an even keel.

7 - Withdrawal

Minimal contact becomes social isolation. Use of psychoactive substances may be used as a coping strategy, like the classic image of an investment-banking high-flier leaving work late to go into the city fueled by cocaine and champagne. The so-called *work-hard, party-hard* attitude. These people may feel directionless and hopeless. Caught in the hamster wheel. Unable to step out and take in the bigger picture, they follow the rat-race week in and week out with scant breaks at weekends. While seeming to be ever involved by being out and being seen to be out, there is no meaningful social engagement or emotional connection as the group colludes with this strategy of isolation in the midst of apparent bonhomie.

8 - Obvious behavioral changes

The changes become ever more apparent to family, friends and colleagues.

9 - Depersonalization

This can be thought of as the first definitive sign. What separates a hard worker from an ill doctor. They lose sight of themselves as someone of inherent worth. They feel like a cog in a machine and cannot see their role as one which is useful. But too scared to withdraw, which should be possible if they are an unimportant cog. Not able to see themselves a vital cog and thus performing a valuable function, they are caught in a no-mans-land, blinkered to any sense of value in the self.

10 - Inner emptiness

The crux. They cannot internally generate self-acceptance and external sources no longer seem effective. They resort to basic biological substitutes to try and release dopamine to replace the absent oxytocin types of experience. Comfort eating and unfulfilling sex are readily available sources of this replacement dopamine surge.

11 - Depression
Symptoms of depression come to predominate with all its biological features. Exhaustion, hopelessness, lack of any perceived meaning in their life and a sense of overwhelming hopelessness.

12 - Burnout syndrome
Crisis point. This needs immediate action as they cannot function any more, physically or emotionally. They may be suicidal as this may seem to be the only way out of the apparently hopeless situation. It is real and not even rare. My local hospital had three completed junior doctor (intern) suicides in the space of two years. I've worked in ten hospitals and rate the work pressures there to be about the median average. Scary stuff.

There are parallels here with developing addictions or hitting the emotional connection pause button to avoid the need to consider one's steady downward spiral of denial. Ways to avoid acknowledging the developing issue such as gambling, substance misuse or having affairs start to surface. Addictive problems and burgeoning burnout can of course run concurrently and confound the issue. It may be that some of these difficulties lead to others and are inextricably intertwined. This would seem to make sense, they can be a presentation of the juggling the needs of the struggling mind and 'sense of an independent self' with the need to influence the world in adverse circumstances. The commonality is that all are probably not very good for you in the long run and are all probably best recognized, possibly explained and then addressed sooner rather than later in order to preserve the precious sense of self and emotional wellbeing.

This is a long list of twelve steps, though not ones that most people think apply to their physicians. It is likely to resonate somewhere for you or someone you know. They cover a vast amount of negative emotion and encompass much of the human capacity to beat oneself up on the inside. It is also deliberately written in a way that nearly everyone will be able to relate to. That isn't necessarily a problem in that it is good to identify with stages of the process as it may help you see things in a different light and hopefully start the process of addressing any reversible negative features and prepare the ground for, or start the journey for moving forward and moving on.

But one also needs to hold in mind the intellectual trap of the horoscope - there is probably a proper term for this. The human tendency to find pattern where there is none. To ascribe meaning where there is none. To link personal applicability when nearly everyone could be linked. It is a an easy mistake to make.

One common cognitive error is to spot it in colleagues and neglect to pay attention ourselves.

Apophenia (G: *apo* = away from + *phaenein* = to show) was coined in the 1950's with **Pareidolia** (G: *para* = alongside + *eidōlon* = image, form, shape) - seeing faces in clouds or holy relics in pieces or burnt toast are fancy terms for this widespread phenomenon. We are pattern seeking creatures. This had an evolutionary selection pressure in that if you see a tiger in the bushes from an indistinct pattern and run away you will live. Whether there was a tiger or not. If you ignore it, then you will be safe most of the time, but get eaten occasionally. So *pattern seekers* over generations had a selective advantage as fewer were eaten.

So just because you think that a lot of the above apply to you - just treat the list with a little caution.

These are simply intellectual prompts, mental nudges. The researchers can of course claim otherwise; their academic prowess, international standing and research grants depend on it. But be circumspect. Take a bigger view. If they did apply to you, how could that be helpful? Is there a way that they could be unhelpful? If so, take a side step and consider a review, a stock check of your current situation. Or ask for help if your brain power is so befuddled you cannot realistically move forward with a clear mind.

Writing stuff down and coming back to it a few days later has a knack of helping sort though these minefields of the mind (Carney and Waters, 2006).

burnout can make you sick

The effects of burnout include health related ones:
- Increase in stress hormones.
- Increase susceptibility to coronary heart disease.
- Depression.
- Cognitive impairment with reduction in nonverbal memory and in auditory and visual attention.

(Sandstrom et al, 2005; Shirom and Melamed, 2005; Patel et al, 2009)

Work absences can be used as a barometer for work satisfaction. A Cochrane review showed that if workers are dissatisfied, feel ill, feel pressured, or undervalued, then absenteeism increases (Ruotsalainen et al, 2014).

Treatment and prevention can be looked at on the level of the individual or that of the organization. This can be further split into the specific workplace factors and the wider healthcare community or nation.

Hatinen et al (2007) talked about the difficulties in addressing the three key symptoms of exhaustion, cynicism and inefficacy. They pointed out that they respond differently to administered preventive or treatment measures.

Exhaustion is more easily treated than cynicism and professional efficacy, which tend to be more resistant to treatment.

There is much research which shows that some interventions can have an adverse effect on performance. This serves as a reminder that individuals must have themselves at the right part of the cycle of change. They have to want to change and be at the right point of acceptance and motivation in that they need to be internally motivated and will not do well if external constraints are imposed or unwanted changes are implemented (Prochaska, 1998).

Not really rocket science, but when we have external constraints thrust upon us, you and I will naturally rebel a bit and won't tend to change as the external person or organization wants us to. Perhaps it is just me. But I do see this in patients with addictions. They will change when they are ready and only then. No amount of extra pressure from a physician before then will produce an effective change (Whitelaw et al, 2000).

The point therefore being that you cannot help someone else move on from whichever of the stages of burnout they find themselves until they are ready. And there may be some careful and sensitive social maneuvering to be done to help nudge them toward that point and allow them to make that next step with your assistance (Van Dierendonck, Schaufeli, and Buunk, 1998).

There is some support for using proactive strategies to prevent burnout (McLaurine, 2008). The research was done in prisons and may not be applicable to medicine. But the feeling among academics is that humans are similar across the board and that work, environmental, social and personal pressures leading to burnout can be extrapolated across professions. Using stress management techniques helps improve employees' stress levels and improves health and wellbeing. Giving employees stress-management tools seems to help too.

Positive features thought to be protective include work commitment, self-directedness and a positive outlook for the future (Elliott et al, 1996).

Again, not much of a surprise, but *sense of autonomy* is an important protective factor (Hätinen et al, 2007).

A combination approach to preventing and managing burnout

in the workplace involves cognitive-behavioral therapy (CBT) and relaxation techniques, both physical techniques and mental. I've included some at the back of this book for your delectation. The Cochrane review by Ruotsalainen et al (2014) found that both organizational and individual level activities may give the biggest gains but getting an organization to change to be more proactive about this sort of thing may well be like trying to relocate a graveyard.

why it matters

Two words: **Morbidity and mortality**. Yours.

Stressed burned out doctors do themselves, their family and just in case you still care; their patients harm.

The serial killer rate among doctors is sky high. They simply top the list of professions: Holmes, Shipman, Swango, Petiot, Ishii, Adams. The list goes on...

We don't know the motivators for these deliberate abhorrent acts. But our collective errors kill people too. By the thousands. We do know that these inadvertent acts or omissions have unwanted consequences and are linked to increased stress levels, spiraling work pressures and burnout (Starfield, 2000; Fahrenkopf et al, 2008; West et al, 2009).

We kill ourselves too. The suicide rate among doctors is embarrassingly and worryingly high. This is not a new problem (Sargent et al, 1977). It is much higher than the general population and has the dubious privilege of topping the charts for professions in some studies (Frank and Dingle, 1999; Schernhammer and Colditz, 2004; Petersen and Burnett, 2008).

Our job is important, yes - but not *that* important. There can't be enough going on in your job to be worth topping yourself over. If that's even on your radar, then things have gone a bit wrong. You yourself and us as a profession need this addressing and sorting out (Worley, 2008; Goldman, Shah and Bernstein, 2015; Schwenk, 2015).

But what about those of us who aren't actually ill or fully burned out? Will we be ok? Not really: Retired doctors in one study lived to be an average 76 years old. My retirement age has just been hiked to 67, with 68 on its way in the next year or two. I don't think the average life-expectancy gives me much cause for celebration (Frank, Biola and Burnett, 2000).

in a nutshell

Where are we at so far? Good question. This is a mental pause page. Take stock.

Are you feeling better yet? Are you hopeful? Is what you're experiencing like a lot of others? Yes? That is a good thing. This burnout problem is real and not about to go away. Feeling validated and understood can be a big step and is an important part of the process of moving forward. So:

- Stop. Take a deep breath.
- Remember that you matter. Also note that probably no one else is going to do it for you.
- Decide to take action.
- Better self-care.
- Again and again.

- Ask for help if you need.
- Don't be afraid to admit a little vulnerability.
- Be professional; are your patients at risk?

I'm not an expert - I'm simply a curator, a fellow traveler. Like a grey haired and friendly museum guide. With a benign smile and a twinkle in my eye, I am here to help steer you. If you know your way around, great. If not - then come inside, I've got a few things to show you that you may like...

You've had or are having a tough time. It's ok for that to feel a bit rubbish. Allow yourself that space. Allow it to sit and just be what it is. Don't try to fight that.

You might like to take time out here, benchmark your situation against some others, ask for some help, re-jig your working day.

Spend some more me-time. Reconnect with loved ones. Read a good novel (or a really trashy one). Come back when you feel a little more human. Renewed and rejuvenated. When you are ready, turn the page.

a vocation

You can't change your job. Can you?

If you can: Do so.

If not then you will need to marshal your resources.

One of the problems with medicine is that society (a bit), our friends and families (a bit more) and we (on some days at least) view the job as a vocation.

A calling. A special calling which affords us rights and privileges to be part of other people's lives when they are at their worst, their most vulnerable. They let us in, they let us help them to the best of our ability.

This is a great burden, a great responsibility but also a great privilege.

This makes being a doctor a little bit special. Because of this we can end up with a bit of a skewed, weird and sometimes very mixed up self-image and become confused about our role both within and without our profession and we can let a lot of things get to us - which no other sane person would allow.

The trouble is that the pressures are so frequent, huge and commonplace that they've become accepted by us, our patients and our families.

But they are doing us harm. They are affecting us… (Charles and Frisch, 2005).

Is there any good news? Well, the first good news is that we can recover from burnout. Secondly, many of us look back at our lives and notice that in years past our mistakes and wrong turnings end up having been opportunities in the making. An unwelcome chance to overhaul various parts of our lives and sometimes we are able to go on to greater and better things. All of which may not have come to pass if we hadn't had the sticky patch which mired us at the time.

While I'm not suggesting that being burned out is a good thing or facing the real risk of spiraling uncontrolled depression is somehow welcome - it may yet turn out to have a silver lining. Forcing your hand to reorganize your physical, mental, and work life can be revivifying.

Ok, I'm clutching at straws to find an upside, but really this *could* have a happy ending.

move the goalposts

There is a story about a man who had borrowed some money from a work colleague. He couldn't afford to repay this debt. As the big deadline approached he lay in bed night after night tossing and turning with worry. In the middle of the night before the debt was due to be paid, his wife, fed up with all the sleepless nights, picked up the phone and rang the colleague. She said:

"He can't afford to pay you. He hasn't got the money. Sorry. Good night."

Turning to her husband she said:

"It's his problem now."

And rolled over and went to sleep.

(Neill, 2009)

Sometimes, moving the goalposts can be helpful. We can end up chasing our own tails into despair and angst over all sorts of things. Sometimes these rules, deadlines, targets, tasks, goalposts and goals are more arbitrary and artificial than we give them credit for.

Try shifting those goalposts from time to time. It can feel very liberating and gives a paradigm shift to the problem. Paradigm shifts with their new perspectives have a knack of presenting solutions that can feel a lot better and let the pressure off.

A paradigm is a model with which we view the world. A useful working framework. Covey (1989) gives an example of a shift he experienced on the subway. Children were running amok while their father did nothing but stare into the distance.

Eventually, compelled to intervene, he demanded of the father that he control the miscreants better. The father raised his head slowly and apologized profusely for their behavior, saying that they were on their way home from the hospital where the children's mother had just died. He said he didn't really know what to think and they probably didn't know how to handle this either. The feelings towards this man flipped in an instant from irritation to compassionate empathy.

Other practical stuff to try:
- Ask for help.
- Accept this help.
- Accept that you are not super-human (at least for *this* week).
- Mix it up and change your environment. (for a minimum of 30 minutes a day; self-pamper, laugh, get out of the house. This change of scenery works like a charm for toddlers as a mental distractor - our wiring is the same even though we are older).
- Share your feelings. Rant at someone. Perform a mental download, this can be cathartic.
- Don't let work be all that you do. Step out from this tunnel vision.
- Find something else that you can attach purpose to. Something which avoids that trap of our identities (as doctors and physicians) being tied up in our job role. When this happens the danger is that we then do not adequately detach from work and thus our downtime is constrained. Which is fine and dandy when things are going well, but when you are burning out you will find it helpful to be able to detach properly.

Strategies for prevention can be categorized as personal and professional. Spickard, Gabbe and Christensen (2002) make some helpful distinctions with suggestions:

Identity:
- Be aware of your core values.
- Have clear goals.
- Be aware if you are a pessimist and consider if a paradigm shift towards optimism could help (the silver lining switch).

Downtime:

- Take adequate care of yourself (eat, sleep, exercise, play).
- Take time out to spend with friends and family.
- Consider spending time in religious activity (this can be any goal-directed, supportive time away from work which aligns with your value system).
- Take time to spend with your significant partner, or do dating to find a new one.

Professional:
- Learn about the locus of control and consider the implications (what you can control, what you can't, to be at peace with the distinction, then try and exert control over only what you can).
- Learn how to say no to stuff you simply have not the time to do well.
- Find a mentor (or become a mentor yourself).
- Use reflective practice (how what you do affects you personally and professionally, look for anything you can celebrate - just occasionally something may go right. Also look for areas you can modify or change to develop your professional role).
- Consider hiring an accountant and a financial adviser.
- Keep your professional development up to date.

Many people find it useful to specifically work on:
- Acceptance - being centered.
- Just being, in the moment.
- Becoming aware of your locus of control
- Looking for a silver lining.
- Taking care of you.
- Sharpen that saw. Benjamin Franklin said that if he had eight hours to cut down a tree he would spend the first six sharpening the saw.

locus of control

Just what is the locus of control? Good question.

Can you control the universe? Would you even want to? That's a lot of juggled balls in the air at any one time and a lot of responsibility. The trouble is, being in control or having this illusion feels good. Being realistic, there is some stuff in our life we can control. And a whole load of other stuff over which we have no influence. There are a few things at the edges that we can sometimes control. Choosing to focus our efforts on things we can control seems sensible. Otherwise there is a whole lot of intellectual, physical and emotional energy which can be expended for little gain. The trick is in working out where these boundaries lie in our own lives. Once we stop trying to change things we can't, life seems to get better. Because when we act on things we can change, we get to change them. And feeling in control feels good.

So the good news here is that we are responsible for our own actions. We get to choose them. Being responsible sounds like it carries all sorts of negative connotations. But I don't think it has to be like that:

Being responsible = Being response **able**.
Able to respond.
Able to act.
Cap**able** of action.

Our locus of control is where we believe the power lies in our life. When the locus is inside us, it feels good and we feel powerful. We are internally directed and feel we are able to make decisions about our own life and choose our own actions. If it seems there is stuff going on in our life that we are trying to control but can't, this doesn't feel good at all. When the locus seems to be outside us, this feels like we are bobbing about on a stormy ocean without any sails or power, left adrift to the mercies of chance (Rotter, 1966).

Being autonomous is a natural driver - this is an urge to be in control which feels good. If we don't feel in control we feel terrible. If we feel in control it feels great (Dormann et al, 2006; Judge, Locke and Durham, 1997).

We spend a lot of time trying to exert our will on the outside world and a lot of time trying to increase that sphere of influence. A lot of stress arises we when try in vain to control stuff we cannot control and in many situations have no realistic chance of ever being able to control. Like the weather, the world economy, events that have already come, been and gone and so on.

If you try to control the universe you will fail. It is a big place.

In medicine we often gain satisfaction from controlling various parameters; we control our work flow, what we say, which medicines to give to which patients and what recommendations to make. This makes sense, it is what we're paid to do and what exactly we've trained for.

Being in control feels good. We feel masters of our own destiny and that of our patients. It feels fine and we get paid to show up and do this stuff. Unfortunately, other people are a bit complex. And unpredictable. You, me, our patients. Annoyingly they don't always do what we want. The pathophysiology isn't always quite like the textbooks and stuff sometimes doesn't work out. As if that wasn't enough, sometimes our employers can't quite see the correct bigger picture like we can. We have to follow their rules, impositions, silly targets and budget restraints. Everyone wants more for less and we can end up shouldering a lot of the blame for this along with the responsibility to fix it. We go out of our way to smooth the troubles and to make the daily wrinkles and challenges disappear. All in the name of trying to provide an ideal standard of excellent care for our patients that perhaps isn't very realistic in the real world.

In the real world chaos theory exists, entropy happens, the universe does its own thing and we are actually in control of very little. Everything else is a convenient mirage, a useful lie. We only really control our own actions, thoughts and the stuff we do, think or say. And if we get right down to it and are really honest we aren't very much in control of those either.

Two choices are to fight this or try in vain to gain every tighter control. Neither are recommended.

The other choice is to take notice of these limitations on our circle of influence and embrace this. It is a fact. This stuff is real. Recognize this for what it is, work with it and move on. Change the stuff you can. Accept what you can't and learn to tell the difference. Whole religions are built on this principle and it's a good one.

I grant you, it isn't always quite that simple or straightforward. It is a bit of an art form to let go of some control. This shifting of the locus of control can take a while to master. But working towards it will bring daily relief from many of our stresses and strains (Benassi et al, 1988; Judge et al, 2002; Park and Searcy, 2012).

All you can do is show up, do the best you can and then reset for the next day. Your best will almost certainly be good enough. If it isn't then take time out, retrain or do some embezzling and move to Hawaii wearing a fake mustache. You *could* get away with it.

Changing the locus of control is helpful (Judge, Locke and Durham, 1997) but change can feel worrying. Even accepting that stuff has gone a bit wrong can be stressful. We are likely to exhibit the characteristic grief reaction phases as we mourn the loss of mentally what we've set up our future to be (Kübler-Ross, 1969).

We are still the same people, with the same bodies, brains, skills and memories but we panic and don't cope well when the future that we had mapped out is taken away by things without our control.

If we plan to change it feels ok and even exciting. When we have it thrust upon us we don't do so well. We deny, become angry, try to bargain and so on. Having the dawning realization that we are burning out and that there are specific helpful steps that need to be taken to bring about progress, healing and recovery can come as a great relief.

But for some of us it can feel pretty rough. It can feel alarming and as if sands are shifting under your feet. If you sense this alarm then follow the wise words from Douglas Adams' *Hitchhiker's Guide to the Galaxy* (1979).

> ***"it has the words DON'T PANIC inscribed in large friendly letters on its cover."***

While the guide you are holding has a significantly less reassuring cover, it will do nicely in its place. Why not close it and take a deep breath. Go for a walk. Enjoy the air. Come back and get ready to move on. We'll wait for you.

pressures

We are all pleasers. We like to be liked. We usually try quite hard to make people like us. The trouble is that other people are fiercely independent and don't tend to do what we want. All rather irksome and a bit of a bore.

Too often we do stuff to try and get the *like-response* in return but other people are mostly up in their own heads, having their own complex lives and don't often give us what we want or need, when we think they should give it. Which feels a little selfish of them. But it ain't going to change just because it isn't very fair on you.

So you can end up working yourself up into tightly wound circles of stress trying to please everyone and getting very little satisfying back. This is not really a very good return-on-investment for all your hard efforts.

Learning to let go of needing this can be tricky. Learning to say no is a crucial part of that. If you have too much on your plate it stands to reason that you won't do all of it. Let alone do it well. Is it really fair on everyone who you are already trying to please or get things done for, to take more stuff on which will inevitably dilute your already stretched and no doubt excellent skills? Saying yes to something when your dance card is filled means giving a poorer result to something you've already got on your list.

Many of us subject ourselves to internal pressures by having impossibly high standards.

It is good to have high standards. We hold ourselves to a high standard of personal and interpersonal conduct. It comes with the job. It goes with the territory. Our patients expect this of us, our professional bodies too; ensuring we act consistently with this by imposing sanctions when we do not.

But this comes at a price. We pay this price internally. We have this ideal we hold ourselves to. This ideal, perfect, professional who never puts a foot wrong, who always learns from their mistakes constructively and readily acknowledges their weaknesses because those all around will applaud them for doing so and think better of them. This perfect person of course never has an off day, they are able to be professional in the face of all and any adversity. Even with budget cuts and incompetent juniors. Even if they have a headache. They can keep their poise consistently, are kind, caring and don't really need sleep or downtime away from the job - as their ongoing professional development should take pride of place in their personal life (Dale and Olds, 2012).

This is of course ridiculous. We sometimes put this ideal up on a pedestal and forget that it doesn't really exist - well, I can't come anywhere close and I hope you are at least aware that some of us can't manage as well as you. This ideal image of a perfect physician is useful. It gives us something to aim for. But we live in the real world, with real problems, with real families and because of this we experience all of life's ups and downs. Just like our patients. To factor in our human-ness is something we can lose sight of.

It is important not to lose sight of this.

learn to say no

You cannot do everything. Your plate is full. You need to curb some stuff and stop accepting more things to do. There are simply not enough minutes in the day to do everything. My inbox has hundreds of items, my to-do list stands over the thousand mark. You may be doing better than me.

Go through your tasks, your piles of paperwork (you do have them too don't you?), your stuff and slash at it with the **80/20 rule**. Do the 20% of your tasks which will bring about the quickest rewards. The rest of it will wait (and eventually may simply become obsolete if you just ignore it long enough).

This is widely accepted as being the Pareto principle. As an undergraduate in economics, the eponymous Vilfredo noted in 19th century Italy that 80% of the land was owned by 20% of the people (Pareto, 1896). Interestingly lots of more stuff in economics turned out to have the same sort of split. It has been extrapolated into myriad fields and specialities as being a truism. It isn't an *actual* law of the universe. It merely states that things get distributed unevenly. And if you pay attention to some of them, effort is best directed carefully to the ones which will bring the best results. So step back and aim your limited resources well. That's all it says. It's still useful today, more than a century on.

We don't have time to do it all. Every day you will have more requests of you and your time than you can possibly achieve in your waking hours. All the stuff you want to do and all the stuff that others want you to do will add up to more than the allocated numbers of minutes in a lifetime.

Of course this assumes you are going to be taking your allotted eight hours of rest each night. And you are: aren't you? That is not really a question. It's a statement. There is no wiggle room on that one. Tempting as it may be to skimp. That would be a false economy. Like building a boat out of paper as it is quicker and cheaper than doing it properly.

So we aren't going to get it all done. What now? Either we relax and accept this, leaving vast swathes of un-performed tasks in our wake or we somehow stem the in-flux of work, jobs and tasks. A dilemma.

The best tool in your arsenal will be the word no. "**No**".

Short, succinct, to the point and can mean many different things in different contexts and intonations; like all my favorite monosyllabic utterances. This can be a very difficult word to say. It comes back to us wanting to please, wanting to keep up a super-human but unrealistic self-image to project to the world.

Learn to say:
"Sorry, if I take this on then I'm going to have to not do something else as my plate is already full. I simply can't do any more right now."

If you keep saying yes, people will keep asking. Once you say no, they will find another way around. You aren't the only human. There are others. Some of these could be given the task. Some may even be quite good at it. But that isn't the point. The point is that *you* cannot take more stuff on.

You are reading this because you are aware of pressures. You need to take charge. The world in general doesn't care very much about you. Sorry about that. The 'you' inside. And you need to look after the internal you. No one else is going to do it and if you don't, who will? Really, who?

So I'm afraid you might have to practice the initially uncomfortable sensation of learning to say *No*. The good news is that acquiring new habits like this are incremental and iterative. They will get easier progressively and predictability so with time. Just like a new pair of shoes. Weird at first, then a little while later and without really noticing, they become your new comfortable shoes which you don't give a second's thought to.

journaling

Not really a proper word. But it will be soon, that's the way language moves on. Evolution of memes, but I digress. When we write stuff down it isn't as fast as the thoughts that flash through our minds. This allows for some organization of the thoughts on the way out. Most people find that very helpful.

I recommended keeping a journal. A collection of thoughts, feelings, ideas and anything else you fancy. I strongly recommend password protecting each document. Then you can write what you like. But do the writing. It really helps.

You never know, you could turn the scrivenings into a book of your own (that's how this one got started).

When we write stuff down we interact with the information on the way out. It is an active process. This active-processing has been shown in learning cognitive science to positively influence retention and integration with existing ideas and concepts to produce new ones (Angela et al, 2012). This is the essence of creativity. No longer is the muse of creativity a formless being who may or not visit. This is the way to harness your inner dormant ideas.

Writing stuff down allows your brain to process this information pre- peri- and post- writing to consolidate old information and produce new thoughts. Merely thinking about this in the abstract or even in the ordered won't produce the same effects. Or at least, not as fast or as effectively (Magdeleine, and Schmidt, 2011).

From a burnout point of view, there will of course be much stuff going on in your brain which you may not want to commit to paper. Edited highlights are acceptable. Consider password protecting your documents or burning them afterwards (most satisfying, but be careful to do this somewhere safe like a basin with readily available running water, far away from pesky smoke detectors. Think: Big Brother).

The point is that the power of actual writing is very much underestimated by those who don't do it. It can of course seem daunting. Many a budding writer and a few experienced ones are paralyzed with fear at the sight of the blank page. The best advice is write to the clock and be prepared to write gibberish. If you can do both those things, then you are away. Don't wait for inspiration to strike. Start at nine o'clock and write for five minutes. Or whatever time you choose. Start with documenting your stream of consciousness, writing down any silly thoughts that crop up. Soon your proper brain will take over and more useful stuff will emerge. You don't have to worry about spelling. You will never show anyone and it is the act itself which is helpful, rather than achieving a cogent output.

Learning journal, dream diary, worry words, stress paragraphs, book ideas, ranting writing - call this what you will. Choose to say whatever you fancy. But try it. Try it today.

Right now. Right here. Write now. Right on. Write on. Alright?

assumptions

I'm guessing that you are not a mind reader.

- Trying to be a mind reader can end you in trouble.
- Remember not to do this.
- Particularly over something which is stressing you. You might just be wrong.

Jaremko and Meichenbaum relate the anecdote:
John's lawn mower broke down and he decided to borrow his neighbor's. As he walked toward the neighbor's house, it occurred to him that his neighbor might not be willing to loan him the mower. This thought appalled him, because he had freely loaned things to his neighbor in the past. The more he thought about how unfair it would be, the angrier he became. When he came to his neighbor's house, he blurted out, "Keep your damn mower. I wouldn't take it if you begged me".
(Jaremko and Meichenbaum, 2013)

"An assumption makes an ass out of u & I."
(Anon.)

Unexamined emotions seem to arise as spontaneous reactions to situations. Cognitive theorists suggest instead that it is the interpretation of the event and not the event itself that causes this emotional response. This means there may be some wiggle room in our reactions. A space to modify what we perhaps had assumed were knee jerk responses over which we have no control.

When we have an emotional reaction that we don't like, aren't keen to show the world or otherwise would like to alter, it seems prudent and sensible to insert a mental pause before reacting. If we can make this habitual, we are then afforded the chance to consider alternative plausible explanations for the events unfolding in front of us. It is in these moments of consideration that our power grows to respond helpfully rather than reacting without thinking.

> *"Engage brain before putting mouth into gear."*
> (my Mum)

I've found that the lawn mower story to be well received by patients as it has enough of a resonance that most of us can relate to.

Our stress levels arise from an imbalance between stuff we have to do and perceived resources to manage these demands. It feels worse when the stakes are higher or the mismatch is greater. If you are handling people's lives in your hands with your every decision and haven't time enough, the manpower, the emotional capacity, the cognitive resources and so on to step up to the plate, then you are going to be feeling it.

If any one of those factors improve you will feel better. If it is a computer game, or you get months to achieve something, or unlimited resources, or a vast, helpful, competent supporting team then it is going to feel better. What sometimes gets overlooked is that the other side of the equation often has some space to maneuver. Sometimes the stakes aren't really going to be fatal in minutes. Sometimes we have more time than we thought or we aren't the only physician in the world at that point in the afternoon who can act.

We are often guilty of making assumptions. I'm guessing you too do this. This isn't always a bad thing. We've evolved strategies for mental short cuts which keep us using optimally low levels of mental power, conserving brain resources. These heuristics enable us to manage to myriad of things we do so excellently, but often uncelebrated, day in and day out for decades of our professional life at a time.

But sometimes these assumptions can be our undoing. Or at least play a part in it. If some of these assumptions are challenged when previously we'd left them alone, they can offer us a lifeline to escape some of the ridiculous and unsustainable pressure that many of us feel all too often.

Some examples:

Our colleagues are all too busy to help.
- What about if I simply ask them?

I must do this today or I am a failure.
- Really? Is there not an emergency number they can call if they get worse before you act? Could someone else with more mental resources actually have more to offer right now? Could you refer elsewhere? And who says you are a failure, others? If so, are they right or simply being mean? Yourself? Why not agree that sometimes you are going to not do everything? Perfectionism is a dangerous thing to juggle. Like pointy knives. All very impressive until you get a little distracted. Or sneeze.

This patient won't listen.
- Perhaps today is the day to negotiate a shared agreement to ask someone else to take a look. A fresh pair of eyes doesn't mean either of you are doing anything wrong. But there are a lot of humans on the planet. Many of whom have differing ideas. Some are just as good as yours. Well, maybe not quite as good, but they will suffice. You get the general idea.

interpersonal conflict

There will be times on our travels through life when we bump up against some other personalities. Inconveniently they can't always see our perfectly reasonable point of view for its patent brilliance.

It can be useful to have some tools in our toolbox for handling these stressful encounters. Gandhi and Socrates had a couple of approaches worthy of mention.

Interpersonal conflicts are ripe in our daily interactions for most of us. When we are tired and feeling the pressure or have burned out we have less resources to marshal in our fight to manage these better. When we have less cognitive capacity we fall back on easier-to-execute mental routines. These leave us open to attack from others.

Here are two ways of engaging the enemy which work, are easy to put into practice and are very effective with minimal input on your part. In short, they give a great bang for your mental buck. We use Socrates and then Gandhi as our two mental hooks.

First up Socrates. This man was a philosopher some two thousand years ago in Greece. He would win a huge proportion of his arguments by getting the opponent to agree with him. Traditionally, arguments were won by presenting your case in a compelling way. Much the same as a TV court room drama has the lawyers addressing the jury with an impressive grandstanding speech filled with dramatic imagery and brilliant lines of reasoning. Socrates used a different method. This became known as Socratic questioning. Ask questions of your adversary to which he can only say yes. Get three yeses and the next thing you deliver will be seen in their head as something they can agree to as well. This gets them on your side without them noticing. Bingo. Job done.

This sneaky technique is used in persuasion engineering by sales people and espoused by Cialdini in his classic *'Influence: The Psychology of Persuasion'* (Cialdini, 1984). The principle of socratic dialog is to elicit agreement to opening statements that your opponent must agree to. You are more likely to get a positive response to subsequent questions (Russell, 1945).

- Do you agree we are both here to move forward or solve this problem? = **Yes**.
- I think you've thought about this deeply and care about the outcome. = **Yes**.
- I wonder if you are wanting the best possible solution here? = **Yes**.
- Will you lend me a twenty? = **Yes**.

Because humans have so many heuristics going on at the same time we can be cunning and exploit these. Salesmen have for millennia figured out effective ways to do just this.

We endeavor to save brain power the whole time. In every waking moment. Most of the time these automated routines run like… well, just like clockwork. They do so very well and our conscious brain pays them no heed. We've honed our individual ones over the decades to suit our environmental niche nicely. This is part of growing up in society. And part of the medical profession. We have lots of automated routines and subroutines which enable us to do our job even when things at home aren't going so well, or if we have a stomach ache, dodgy bowels and a whole range of other distractors.

Our patients also have these autopilots and books are filled with cunning strategies for allowing us to sidestep and utilize these for the power of good. It is quite beyond the scope of this book (and probably its author) to unveil them here.

Next up is Mohandas Karamchand Gandhi (1869 – 30 January 1948) and his famous story as the underdog Indian lawyer who pretty much single handedly brought down the mighty British empire with his leading by example of non-violent resistance to the British occupation of India.

Famously he would try to visualize all the points of view of the argument. And by doing so, could pre-empt what all his opponents would be thinking and thus their strategy and thereby have prepared suitable rejoinders to anything they might say in public debate or the courtroom.

Exploiting his empathic understandings, he would then use their viewpoints to be able to argue from the adversaries angle, taking the proverbial rug from under them, making himself seem more powerful and better prepared by comparison, elevating his standing and furthering his steady but relentless progress and single aim of removing the British from what he declared to be their illegal occupation of his homeland.

So your two techniques are:

One - to get your opponent to agree with you and your proposition by getting the *yes set*.

Two - be empathic. Argue everything from their point of view. They cannot help but agree as you set out your desired outcome couched in their language and from their angle.

we are pleasers

Many of us became doctors because we wanted to help people. Helping others feels good. The human law of reciprocity gives us a biological drive and a genetic imperative to help others (Pinker, 1999). It aligns with many moral codes and is enshrined in most of the world religions' teachings.

We like to help and we like to be thought of well. Our standing within our social group has this powerful biological driver and our psychological wellbeing depends on it. Our hunter-gatherer group is no longer well defined but social reputation and peer group opinions continue to exert a powerful effect in the twenty first century.

If we aren't careful, we will tend to agree to more stuff than we can realistically handle well. All in an effort to please people, to not to let others down (in our own minds) and to try and curry favor (frequently sub-consciously).

The difficulty here is that being physicians, we are often in positions where we could potentially do a lot of things for a lot of people. Because of this we tend to get asked often to do more than is practical or reasonable.

We want to please, so don't often turn away requests. This ends up being our downfall. It is crucial to monitor and then marshal our finite resources. Budgets, time, mental energy, emotional energy and the logistics of trying to be in more than one place at a time all need to be taken care of.

All too easily they start to spiral out of control. The most important patient is you. Look after this one well and the rest will get better care.

being human

On being human: You are.

There, I said it.

You cannot work effectively if you are not feeling great.
You cannot feel great if the pressure is too great.
You cannot work well when you are ill, tired, hungry or have not got enough emotional support.

Being human has some downsides. You will need some TLC. It isn't *all* bad, there are some good sides too. The world has got a lot of nice stuff in it, if we would only stop and notice it once in a while.

As you haven't got your super-powers turned on, you will need to take stock, marshal your resources (yes, I'm like a broken record) and take a positive stance in order to face the universe and all it has to throw at you:
- Draw lines in the sand. A special circle around your little domain. You can change it later and your circle may grow. But you need first to say *'Stop. This is where I'm at.'*
- Learn to say no.
- Learn to say it in a way that is congruent with your outlook on life (see above).
- Learn that saying no to this means saying yes better to something you've already agreed to. You can justify most things this way, which is handy as our internally generated desire to be consistent is a super-powerful drive and will need to be satisfied.

Next, reduce your job stress. It would be lovely if our employers were to recognize what is going on and change the externally generated pressors to give us space to breathe, support to grow and nurture our recovery and subsequent growth. Clearly this would be efficient and would lead to increased productivity overall, along with our happiness as a happy coincidence.

But this is the real world and everyone is so tied up in their own little world of stress that no one will notice us and still less care. Healthcare organizations are likely to be similarly myopic, with an eye on their employees' health and the ideal of having a sensible eye on future workforce planning only existing in a land of unicorns.

So it is up to you and me to sort this out ourselves. Don't expect much help. Ask, sure. Tell them in a big clear voice where your boundaries are, but expect that it'll take a while to get the buggers to listen. They are institutionally deaf.

Being human brings some personal bits which aren't helpful but can be shifted. Like a new pair of shoes. They will feel odd when you first start to change them, but they can, do and will get better. Do them every day. Work on these.

Here are some to consider:

Stop trying to be so perfect. You will never win. 'Satisficing' is a term which means that *it* is enough. Good enough for today's job. Sure, strive to be great. This is a good thing. But sometimes you just need to get the thing out there. This will then allow to you tinker later or to do better next time. Stressing about the tiny details and never getting the task finished or beating yourself up once it is done will not help your overall day. Learn to let go a little. Do your best in the moment. No one can ask more of you.

Also if you are perfect, you are going to annoy your colleagues. The perfect ones annoy me. In the interests of a harmonious workplace, allow others to see you as not quite god-like. They will warm to you faster. If you are pretty perfect it is probably best to keep that to yourself!

Turn up on time. Leave on time. Leave extra commute time if you need. There will always be a need to find a parking space. Leaving an extra three minutes early and driving at the speed limit takes the same time and you arrive feeling tranquil. Don't listen to the morning news. The extra gain in social currency is minimal and it mostly contains stories of how dreadful the economy is, terrorism, wars, calamities and natural disasters or unimportant political or celebrity gossip which won't matter much in five years. Consider going on a news diet (ingest no news for a month).

Run to time. Be tidy, de-clutter. Answer all messages and emails the same day. Clear your in-tray. Have a one-touch office. This will de-clutter your brain by decreasing the number of balls you feel you are juggling. The key to this is quick brief interventions and delegate, delegate, delegate and keep really clear electronic notes you can access anywhere. Review these often and mercilessly cull the stuff you aren't going to do. It can always go back on the list later.

Look for the silver lining. If you are like the chicken who thinks the sky is falling you will have a rubbish day. It may well fall but you can't control that. Back to the locus of control. Exert your influence over the stuff you *can* affect. Look for the positives and life will actually feel better (Lyubomirsky and Layous, 2013).

It's worth learning to reverse engineer your brain - put that smile on with every patient. Sit up straight, lean forward. Smiling and leaning forward looks positive, comes across well and on the inside actually feels good. Turn down the voice of your internal dialog. Every patient encounter is an opportunity to help someone. That is quite a special privilege. And few people get this chance multiple times a day. We are pretty lucky. Even if you cannot change the dismal outcome of a patient. Knowing that you've listened and really heard them, makes them feel better about it. Do this.

Locus of control includes not controlling other people. What they do, think, say or how they choose to live their life is their decision to make and you have to let them. Use the **god-mantle** of traffic calming as a guide (we'll come to this). Don't let any of your happiness depend of what they do. That is the path to stress and sadness. Because mostly they are buggers and don't do what you want. This challenge is at least as old as King Cnut (990-1035AD) and the apocryphal failure to control the tide. We laugh at the popularly mistold story now - but is this sometimes you? I know I'm like this often and the more I can let go, the better. A bizarre upshot of this is that the more you let go, the better you feel and this is rather contagious People actually then start to behave in the way you want. I'm not sure if this is the halo effect, self delusion or something else entirely. But it is nice to notice and improves one's day further.

I know you are human but sometimes it is fun to pretend otherwise. The next time you are in slow moving traffic, feeling all grumpy at the morons who surround you, pop your '*god-mantle*' on. Pretend to be a super-natural being with all the powers that go along with the job. Rather than feeling anger at other road users, you may start to feel pity. It isn't their fault. They are like stupid insects who think they are important, but you know better. Their tiny brains are as nothing to you and you could squash them or send a lightning bolt in their direction if the mood took you. But because you are a wise and benevolent god, you instead choose to spare their pitiful, meaningless lives. You smile benignly and allow your mind to wander to more important higher things as you let the stress of these idiots simply wash away.

Well, it works for me sometimes.

we cannot be seen to be weak

Most of us have been brought up in a machismo culture which allows for no external show of weakness.

We were encouraged to be competitive at school to be in a position to apply for medicine. We then competed with our classmates with our exams being scored and ranked according to performance. We then competed and vied for the top jobs on leaving and this competition continued all the way through the junior intern years to the top consultant and attending jobs or most desirable primary care posts.

During this competition we had to have a game-face which belied no inner doubt. No uncertainty. We were not encouraged to show any lack of knowledge. Our patients, we learned, want us to be strong, to be there for them, to be knowledgeable and always able to help.

Very few of us are encouraged to show our vulnerability, our frailty, our human-ness. Many of the world's leading journals carry a hint of the strength of the soft side. They publish pieces on art, a few poems, a few reflections about the benefits of a human connection with our patients. But this has never caught on properly. No spreading of this by wildfire. It sits consigned to the back pages. An unimportant curious afterthought.

The problem stems from the fact that these weakness and frailties affect us all but they are not discussed. The elephant sitting big and obvious in the corner of the room. They are not aired. We seem expected culturally as physicians to sail through life as an elegant swan. There is an unspoken understanding that underneath we are paddling like crazy just to stay in one place. But few talk about it.

Probably none of your peers would tell you about how the workload sometimes reduces them to tears and the pressures can have them crying in the car not wanting to emerge. Or that sometimes they lock themselves in the bathroom for longer than they need to so they don't have to face whatever they have next.

It is these things of which we dare not speak. We don't ask for help. No one usually offers to help. We dare not ask for the fear of seeming weak.

This is probably a mistake and built on a lot of assumptions about ourselves and other people which may not be true. Exposing a soft underbelly is dangerous in combat or in the wild. But in medicine - it might not have any consequences at all except that perhaps your colleagues and friends may be more understanding and may even offer to help. It is just possible. They may even and with a tear in their eye proclaim: *'me too.'*

we cannot be ill

We are not allowed to be human. No one can see that we are people with flesh, blood, desires, weaknesses and flaws, just like our patients.

What if we were to discovered? To be found out. To be uncloaked as not actually perfect, omniscient and immortal. What then? What if they realize that our thin veneer of expertise is nothing more than a lot of experience, training and carefully applied knowledge.

Surely that unveiling of the magic trick by pulling back the curtain will in one fell swoop cause all our patients to lose faith? If the mystery of the faith healer is lost, we will surrender our power and the shimmery luster of our shiny cures will fade when exposed to the full bright morning sun.

Well, err, maybe. But modern medicine is different. It is evolving as the role of the clinician is changing. Nearly daily.

No more are we the infallible fount of knowledge espousing clever stuff from our pedestal. We don't make patients cower and grovel. We don't make them bow and scape as they leave the consultation. Well I don't when I think anyone else might be looking.

We are more curators now. The librarians who lead people to find stuff out for themselves. We help them make sense of all the information out there. And there is a lot. This is a good thing. It takes the pressure off us a bit. We no longer have to know it all. This is also a good thing.

But it can be a bit of an ego-dent when you first try to get your noggin around this.

I trained initially as a surgeon. Trying vainly to ape the attitudes of my seniors. My ego was huge. My empathy and compassion zero. I was of course an insufferably arrogant idiot and pretty annoying to be around, let alone talk to. And very very wrong. Unknown unknowns as popularized by Joseph and Harrington in the Johari window (Luft and Ingham, 1955). I didn't know much and had not enough social skills to be able to spot that. Over the last few years I've gained an eye-watering amount of insight and it is still very much a painfully awkward work in progress (this book clearly isn't offered from a point of knowledge and arrogance, elevated from a dais, but more out of a kinship of admitted foibles, compound errors and personal weaknesses).

Can you be ill? I would say: *Hell yeah!* And you should 'fess up when you are: Seek help and support. It should be readily available. If it isn't, stomp your feet until it is.

Your profession, colleagues and friends alike have a duty of care not only to their patients but to each other. And this includes you. We all do. We have to remain vigilant.

> **"*Quis custodiet ipsos custodes?*"**
> (Juvenal and Escott, 2015).

This Latin phrase from the Roman poet Juvenal in his Satires (Satire VI, lines 347–8) is literally translated as: *"Who will guard the guards themselves?"*

For docs, we need to look after one another - both as a supportive network and as patients.

We all want to do good by using our magical healing powers (see above) and we should do the greatest good for the greatest number of people (Beneficence - one of the *prima faciae* standard ethical principles put forward by Beauchamp and Childress, 1979).

We thus have an imperative need to heal the physicians first - this makes those practising more effective and if we help those not currently able to practise, we get more functioning physicians on the ground and at the front line to minster our benevolent white magic to the populus.

you are not a robot

This, inconveniently for some, means you have feelings.

Feelings are good, they make us feel human. Having an emotional response to events in the outside and the inside world is normal. It doesn't always feel good though.

To be an effective physician, we have to tread the delicate tightrope between compartmentalizing patients and thus allowing for sensible, dispassionate, careful and rational decisions. And empathizing with patients and feeling what they feel in order to be able to understand, care and to share with them a fragment of their journey. This human compassion is something which many patients tell us brings solace and comfort in their illness. Cutting through the modern science and the unpleasant treatments, this human connection is something that for many of us embodies just what it is to be a caring physician.

But care too much, let too many people in and you will inevitably start to crumble. There is just too much suffering out there and too many tragic human stories for us to engage with them all. Whom do you choose? Do you let them choose you? Where do you set your boundaries? When do you relax your professionalism and allow human connections in?

These are not easy questions and extended discussions with definitive answers are well beyond the scope of this tome. This book is supposed to be a helpful guide only. I raise this only because these feelings are common. I most often hear them discussed with doctors in training as they are coming upon these weighty topics afresh and not surprisingly feel that they can loom, large and scary.

Clarifying questions, is this me?
- Do you find yourself even at the beginning of the week longing for the weekend?
- Are you in a funk?
- Have you lost your mojo?
- Are you permanently tired, unmotivated and clock watching?
- Do you find yourself avoiding people or certain work tasks?
- Could you represent your country at the international procrastinator games? They are real, but no one has yet got around to organizing the next venue.
- Do you snap at your spouse, colleagues or children?
- Do you patients wind you up?
- Are you left at the end of the week with a huge pile of tasks and that overwhelming sensation that there's never enough time to get everything done?
- Do you feel empty and like the whole thing (your life, medicine) is a complete waste of time?

The Harley levels are about covering the basics; body mind and spirit:
First **feed yourself** then rest yourself (body).
Mind next - quieten it. Slopey shouldered, get rid of your work pressures. Ask for help and unplug.
Spirit - this regenerates (motivation, like bathing is needed daily). Handily each morning hope regenerates.

There is a biochemical basis for mentally decluttering. Effortful thinking actually needs more energy. Vital glucose consumption by your cerebrum (Kahneman, 2012). Emotional stuff, likewise.

Stuff in your life which is stressful uses up these energy stores (as measured by stroop tests). They decrease like a phone battery each day. Which is why snacking destroys diet plans most evenings despite your morning efforts.
- making effortful decisions becomes progressively more tricky towards the end of the day. Harder to take the long view and easier to hit the *here and now* instant gratification button.
- when you have competing modules and motivations in your brain, the more complex decisions will do worse as the day

wears on. Meaning whatever you have ingrained into habitual behavior will win out.
- nightly proper recharge is needed or you take this on over into the next day.

Basics = food + water + sex + sleep + emotional connection + support and love.
Work on these. Ignore them at your peril.

A handy shortcut to get started is to move the goalposts, to lower your standards. Drop your ideals - this is a good way to rapidly make your daily stuff feel a bit easier. You don't really have to compromise who you are. But just try it on for a few days. Again - just like a new habit, doing this will inevitably feel uncomfortable. If it does, then you probably are trying quite hard enough. If is feels easy and you aren't bumping up against the edge of your comfort zone (where the magic of change in self-improvement actually starts to happen), push further. You will like the results.

If you don't, you will at least gain valuable insight (*I don't fail, I only gain feedback* - empirical epistemology) - write these down, reflect on your experience. This is learning log and reflective journal gold. Your revalidation and professional body live to see this type of reflective practice. It's also a fabulous insurance for if things go belly-up to show you have insight and have at least have *tried* to do something about it - even is that something was too little, too late, not enough, not the right something or was aimed a little in the wrong direction.

Did I mention that delegating is good? Winston Churchill (1874-1965) is frequently attributed with:
"Delegation is the art of leadership."

Delegate, delegate, delegate.

Then delegate some more. Then go home - you've done enough for the day.
- triage, triage, triage (from the French *trier* = to sift).
- do the important urgent stuff.

- then delegate.
- then go home and cover your basics (rest, recuperate, recharge your body, mind and spirit).
- come back, crack on, use Pareto's 80/20 to slash at your tasks, triage and delegate some more.
- again and again.
- then rest and recharge.

Rinse and repeat. You get the general idea.

This is the start of the new you. How exciting.

the human physician

Being human carries its needs.

The upside is that it is this very human-ness which allows us to connect. To empathize. To understand our patients. To be able to glimpse their journey, to be able to see, if only briefly, the world through their eyes.

It is in this fleeting emotional connection and shared understanding that we are able to be at our most effective. What seems the best course of action from your point of view sometimes seems absurd to the patient in front of you.

By being able to recognize your limits and the limits of what modern medicine can do, you are able to join them in making the best decisions and treatment plans.

Your weak side is part of you. It is this very weakness that is one of your strengths as a physician.

Now, how to stop your weak side making your whole working life an unremitting nightmare. We face this challenge when avoiding or recovering from burnout.

When facing someone else with an unreasonable (*id est* not your) agenda:
- Step back, take a bigger picture.
- Does this REALLY matter?
- Don't send back grumpy messages.
- Don't lash out.
- Bite your tongue (try not to bite off someone else's).
- Try and work out if the other person is hating you / just a moron / simply tired and pursuing their own crazy ideas. And

remember, if they are a moron it isn't really their fault.
- Either man up and ride above it - or treat it as a training issue and try to explain kindly (treat them like a petulant but stupid two year old - while elegantly making them feel special and not like you are patronizing them, which means talking down to them, which of course you are, but be artful and don't let them spot it).
- The world is full of morons who can't mindread your excellence and haven't yet cottoned on to your blatantly obvious brilliance and have the near-sighted temerity to question your plans.
- Learn instead to be god-like and rise above the nonsense they throw in your face (be they politicians, reporters, the public, patients and even dareisay esteemed colleagues from time to time).
- Develop a serene god-complex and gain some pleasure from each time you exercise your god powers and are able to not react and can sort out the situation without denouncing the offending party as a dunderhead in public. They may be a dullard, but informing them is unlikely to help and you can get better results by doing it yourself or cascading education their way.
- An even better strategy is to loudly **'big them up'** in public, proclaiming them to others as excellent, thus forcing them to try and live up to the brilliant reputation that you've constructed on their behalf. This is surprisingly effective and ticks all the boxes above (I grant you it can be a bit tricky at first to metaphorically bite your tongue when all every fiber in your body want to simply scream at them and beat your head, or theirs, against the desk while weeping tears of bitter frustration). They may of course be simply having a bad day and bawling them out won't improve their woefully lacking coping capacity. If this is the case, buy them a copy of this book (&/or a chocolate bar) and do the above steps anyway.

Because you are human, you can become ill too. Sorry about that, but there you go. Stress is normal but doesn't make you ill. Not nice but a part of life. Burnout is when the stress has gone on for far too long and you've become dysfunctional. But it can be masquerading for something different. You could *actually* be ill. Mental and or physical illness may coexist. Do not overlook whether you could have a real physical condition which needs prompt attention. You are a qualified physician, so do not neglect symptoms or signs. This does not make you a hypochondriac. It reveals you to be smart.

A hypochondriac is at a party. The lights go out. Everyone cries out:

"What happened to the lights?"

The hypochondriac cries out:

"My eyes, what's happened to my eyes?"

When to seek professional help:
- Don't forget physical illnesses. Seek help if this applies to you.
- When you think you need some formal mental health involvement. Seek early help. It is better to be safe than sorry.
- When what you are doing isn't enough or you are sliding, take advice.
- Seek a doctor if you aren't sure. Talking therapies can be extremely therapeutic and you are intelligent enough to get something out of pretty much any counselor out there, so find a cheap one.

If you are *really* struggling, then hire a reputable, more expensive one. Doctors are bright and solution focused, so often respond really well to a cognitive behavioral therapy type approach (Guille et al, 2015). CBT is based on about twelve sessions, usually with homework to do in-between. There are therapists out there who specialize in just this. Seek out and engage their services.

Making progress and starting to heal yourself may be as simple as opening yourself up and then asking for help, which is the biggest most significant step. Not always the easiest, but important nonetheless. Simply acknowledging you are fallible, vulnerable and then asking for help goes a long way to rectifying a dismal situation.

you are not a machine

You are not a machine either.

This means you need your rest, sleep, feeding and adequate downtime.

This is common sense. But as Voltaire noted in his 'dictionary philosophique' - common sense isn't actually all that common:

> *On dit quelquefois: "Le sens commun est fort rare."*
> People sometimes say: "Common sense is quite rare."
> (Voltaire, 1765)

The problem of burnout is all pervasive, a pandemic. Research from the city health department in Guangzhouin China showed 39% of doctors and 61% of nurses had psychological problems, working an average of 46.4 hours a week, with 17% having suicidal thoughts (Dayi, 2008).

In India the news is grim: Dr Sarda from Pune told the Indian Medical Association that an analysis of IMA's social security scheme of 11,000 doctors showed the average lifespan of a doctor in India to be 55-59 years, while an average Indian lives up to 69-72 years (Sarda, 2016).

In Japan things are apparently better, but not by much. They Graduate at 25.17 with a future life span of 52.88 years. Giving a life span of 78.05. That is about forty one years of work and then eleven years of retirement (Nishi et al, 1999). Is that a fair exchange?

We are not only killing ourselves, but our patients too. It seems no one is safe. Dr Barbara Starfield published in the JAMA

(2000), finding that iatrogenic deaths are the third leading cause of mortality in the United States resulting in the loss of 225,000 lives per year. Broken down into:
- nosocomial infections = 80,000 dead.
- physician errors = claim 27,000.
- unnecessary surgery = 12,000 killed.

This study doesn't suggest a causal link to this culling of warzone proportions but it doesn't stretch the epidemiological mind too much to find a mental association with stress and burnout. Errors are far more common in burned out physicians (Fahrenkopf et al, 2008; West et al, 2009). I'm sure I make less errors on a good day (fewer, dammit).

A study of obituaries published in the British Medical Journal (Patel et al, 2009) found that doctors who qualified in the developed world appeared to live longer (mean age at death of 78 years) than those who qualified in Asia (mean age at death of 70 years). With White-European doctors living significantly longer than doctors from other ethnic groups. Those numbers all sound rather early to me. But worse was to come: An eighth (12.5%) of doctors died between the ages of 60 and 70 years and, of these, nearly half died between the ages of 61 and 65 years. The authors stated that:

'Retirement at ages of 65 years or above would disadvantage nearly one in six medical practitioners.'

I think 'disadvantage' somewhat understates this.

They concluded that cardiologists are not immortal, succumb in their early seventies and need to retire gracefully as early as is currently permitted. Wise words indeed.

But doctors aren't really an unhealthy bunch, are we? Frank, Biola and Burnett (2000) wrote about mortality rates and causes among U.S. physicians. They died at: 73.0 years for white and 68.7 for black. They concluded:

'These findings should help to erase the myth of the unhealthy doctor. At least for men, mortality outcomes suggest that physicians make healthy personal choices.'

I'm not sure I'm happy with that. My current retirement age in the UK is set by the government, sitting currently at 67. It is being suggested that it will shortly become 68. That's getting a bit close for comfort.

sleep

'Sleep is the breakfast of champions.'
(Dr Phil Harley)

Originally Wheaties held the top position as was proclaimed on 'Wheaties' packets from 1927. The iconic crunchy, corn-based breakfast cereal was launched in 1922 and is indeed yummy. But I think the scientific benefits of adequate nightly shut-eye just edges it.

Sleep is where we recharge. More is known today about sleep than ever before and the unearthed findings have surprised many (Benington and Heller, 1995; Spiegel, Leproult and van Cauter 1999; Belenky et al, 2003; Carney and Waters, 2006; Stickgold and Matthew, 2007; Knutson and van Cauter, 2008; Gallicchio and Kalesan, 2009; Ferrie et al, 2011).

While our conscious brain shuts down and our bodies go into rest and repair mode, our brains are anything but quiet.

Our brains busy themselves filtering, filing and storing the day's events. Synapses strengthen and pathways scintillate, finding connections to prior experience and making meaningful sense of the billions of pieces of sensory information that have arrived over the previous day.

It is during sleep that the brain quietly sorts through its problems, it comes up with creative new solutions, it deals with difficult emotional issues and is able to take a meta-view of the day's events to put them into perspective.

"People often say that motivation doesn't last. Well, neither does bathing - thats why we recommend it daily."

(Zig Ziglar, motivational speaker)

We wake afresh with renewed hope, optimism and enthusiasm. We feel recharged and ready to face the next day with its own special challenges and opportunities.

Well, sometimes.

It too often depends on the number of hours and the quality of the sleep we are able to achieve. Getting good quality and an adequate quantity of sleep is crucial, but too many of us skimp on this vital aspect of mental health and wellbeing in the mistaken belief that we are achieving useful stuff by staying up late or trying to burn our precious life-candle at both ends.

Sleep well. I mean it. Do everything you can to secure deep, restful sleep for all the needed hours each and every night. For most of us this means eight hours while it is dark. If you'd like some pointers, these tips are evidence based and effective:

- Avoid alcohol and chemical sedatives - they will blunt optimal crucial frontal lobe activity.
- Be comfortable and feel safe.
- White noise works well (YouTube.com has many excellent files). Blackout blinds can be effective too.
- As we become more senior, don't forget the bladder actions. You won't sleep well if you rise to wee hourly. These bladder pressures are predictable and can be adjusted as your bladder sensitivity can be trained to an extent. Micturate before bed and go easy on the fluids after 17h00 (not a typo).
- There is polyphasic sleep (predominantly bi-modal). If you wake naturally after four hours; panic not. Rise, urinate, read quietly for thirty to sixty minutes and return to bed for your remaining four hours. Some people seem to do this preferentially.
- Consider daytime naps. They have a restorative effect.
- Downtime should lead into sleep.
- In the evening, one should avoid the blue spectrum of light if getting off to sleep is an issue (basically this means no smartphones, TV, computer or tablet devices). The blue light

issuing from the screens mimics morning light and confuses your pineal gland and your inbuilt circadian rhythms.
- Learn the progressive relaxation stuff (handy exercises are to be found in the appendix - not yours, I mean at the end of this book).
- Keep a dream diary.
- Use your 'going to sleep' thoughts as a deliberate worry-then-relax phase. Keep a written list of the stuff that plays on your mind. Your brain has a knack of sorting through this and making progress while you are gaining valuable shut-eye.
- Rise at a set time.

Right, that's enough for now. I need a nap.

downtime

What is your downtime?

Are you thriving with this - or hitting a mental snooze alarm?

These are good questions. We will now look for the answers. If you are zoning out - is there a better, more constructive way to do this? How many chemicals are you using to escape? Are you really helping yourself here the best way you are able? Would you recommend that to a patient?

Are you getting enough physical movement done during each day to give your muscles and cardiovascular system an effective daily workout? Zumba, salsa, jogging, rowing (I mean with an ergo or out on the water, not with your partner), cycling or skiing. Sex counts too, which is nice (that can be with your partner). We are designed to be active for hours and hours at a time, each and every day.

Look at animals (furry, not party animals), they conserve energy when they need to. But daily they run, jump, climb and participate in play activity even as adults. This is inbuilt, it seems smart for us not to neglect these apparently vital activities.

Physicians are largely sedentary, we do wander about - but the heart rate doesn't rise and we don't really do breathless sweaty stuff at work. Well I don't.

It is this effortful movement which maintains our muscles and keeps our VO2 max up - this gives us the neurochemical drivers for better mental health and staves off the rising obesity which so many of seem to have caught - perhaps from our patients?

If your downtime is optimized and you are still burning out, is your work routine to blame? What else could be the root cause that might be usefully attended to?

Your work pattern can be the cause of burnout:
- *poor locus of control.*
- *poor reward structure and lack of recognition for efforts.*
- *under and overwhelm from workload.*

Your lifestyle can lead to burnout:
- *too much work, too little play.*
- *taking on too much.*
- *inadequate downtime and sleep.*
- *not enough social, emotional or family support.*

You on the inside could have predisposing factors:
- *being a perfectionist (that should really read; the need for precision or even being pernickety).*
- *being a pessimist.*
- *being a control-freak.*
- *saddled with the glory of being a high achiever and general aweseomness.*

Could this actually be an esteem issue with the need for externally generated approval? Being a perfectionist can render this approval as never being enough as how do we ever *really* know the approval is warranted, valid, or real; so the cycle continues of every further striving.

Everyone needs some approval. Where you get it is one of the keys to work and personal happiness and general wellbeing. Internals may survive better than externallers. Internally generated approval can be seen to be egotistic: 'I'm so great'. But it's not all bad - if you are able to hold onto this feeling and not therefore need to prove yourself to others this can generate a lot of happiness and a sense of abundance.

If you can be externally humble and manage this with humility, you are a yogi master. If one can maintain this facade but have a psychopathic personality, not really caring about others, this can shine through. One appears like 'Gordon gecko' and people typically think that person is a bit of a knob.

If you rely on externally generated feedback you run the risk of feeling you are never quite good enough and become a people pleaser, which is exhausting and puts you at the mercy of people who frequently turn out to be knobs who care not one whit about you.

If you one who thrives on externally generated inputs and get the right support, you do well. But you are a delicate little flower and are at mercy of not being watered and not being adequately sheltered. Both of which are often out of your control. Being a precious snowflake is all very pretty, but does you no favors.

Learning how and when to shift your locus of control can help. The further in the better. This then allows your influence over the external world to spread.

feeding

"If you don't eat, you die."

(Confucius, attrib.)

True enough. But putting the wrong fuel in does not help you to live well. We are onmivores and are well adapted to eat everything. We are adept at extracting the required nutrients from pretty much anything we shove in the top end. But surviving and thriving are at different levels. As published by Abram Maslow (1943).

Nutritionally speaking, are you helping yourself?
- *Is your diet a high quality diet?*
- *Are you snacking on the go?*
- *Is what you eat really healthy?*
- *Do you need that many carbs?*
- *Are you getting fatter?*
- *Do you feel sluggish?*
- *Do you need to be a little more proactive?* Too often we run out of minutes in the day for food preparation as we feel this steals from what little free time we do have. We then rebel and have a big blow-out meal because we feel we deserve it. While this may be true, is it helpful?
- *How often do you eat until it hurts?*

All our working days are pressured and we all have routines to help us cope. Many of them could be tweaked a little to improve the outcome.

Our stomachs can feed us false information. They would love to be perpetually full so we don't die from lack of sufficient calories. The message is loud and clear - you could die. Eat as much as you can. We base our grazing around these false premises. But we are not at risk of imminent starvation. We aren't about to run out of calories any time soon, so we don't need to snack. Ever. Really. Being hungry isn't fatal and it doesn't even dent concentration or mental activity. What would be the biological evolutionary selection pressure in stopping you thinking clearly when hungry? Your brain needs to be in gear to hunt. Anything less than full throttle mental capacity would be selected out by failing to hunt and gather effectively. It might not always feel like this - but it makes sense. Basically, you do not need snacks. Ever.

Caffeine can be used - but do this judiciously. You don't want to get into the vicious cycle of feeling tired, have lots of caffeine, caffeine still in bloodstream at bedtime, not sleeping well with palpitations (extrasystoles, plus awareness of increased rate and stroke volume), then feeling unrested come the morning, then feel the need for extra caffeine that day and so the cycle goes around. Cumulative sleep deprivation is dangerous and caffeine does not obviate this risk (Belenky et al, 2003; Brown et al, 2009; Gallicchio and Kalesan, 2009).

Eating behavior affects weight and thus the development of obesity. Stress affects this too, as does adequate sleep (Knutson and van Cauter, 2008; Scheer et al, 2009). Studies on the effect of occupational burnout (exhaustive fatigue, cynicism and lost occupational self-respect caused by chronic work stress) on eating behavior are lacking. Though Nevanpera et al (2012) did show that women experiencing burnout at baseline had significantly higher scores in emotional eating (EE) and uncontrolled eating (UE) than did those without burnout. Uncontrolled eating was higher in those with burnout. They concluded:

"Those experiencing burnout may be more vulnerable to EE and UE and have a hindered ability to make changes in their eating behavior. We recommend that burnout should be treated first and that burnout and eating behavior should be evaluated in obesity treatment."

Not really a surprise. A reasonable conclusion. But it is nice that the data is real.

So, be warned. Be careful. Do stuff with forethought, planning and awareness. Especially planning your fueling strategy. While addressing burnout directly, perhaps attack the challenge at both ends and learn to savor. Savoring food and eating more slowly is associated with better weight control. The **20, 20, 20 rule** works surprisingly well for weight loss and waist management (each forkful being the size of a **twenty** pence piece or a quarter, chew each mouthful **twenty** times and eke each meal out for a full **twenty** minutes). This works. You're welcome.

being whelmed

Hitting the sweet spot of busy-ness in our lives can be a challenge.

It is all too easy to take on too much. If we then offload any or all of this - we become restless and bored. Aim to be whelmed. Not over whelmed. Not under whelmed. Just whelmed.

Analogy: you are a little like a **tiger**…

You are fundamentally beautiful.
Magnificent to behold.
Need a great diet.
Get grumpy if people get in your way.
Not much fun to be in front of if you lash out.
Can be tamed, but only by someone really skilled.
Don't like being caged.
Like your freedom.

You also:
- Need time to wash and groom yourself.
- Need to have fun stuff to hunt.
- Hunting can be tricky, that's ok.
- Your prey shouldn't be too small or boring .
- Ready made meals provide no challenge.
- Like to hang around mainly with other tigers.
- Although lions are in the same big family, you probably won't hang around together, That's ok, no one expects you to.
- If you kill indiscriminately people aren't going to be impressed. Even if you are having a bad day, they aren't going to accept that as an excuse.
- If you kill and then eat or otherwise dispose of the body, it still counts. Unless you aren't caught.

There is, I appreciate a limit to this analogy, but the point is: you are fabulous just the way you are. No need to change. But you do need to feel free and you need to allocate time for self-care and enough adequate exercise. Grrr.

multi-tasking

Multi-taking well is a myth. No one can do it effectively. We can all do more than one thing at a time, but we don't do it well. None of us do. Or can. Trying in vain to do this wastes times, energy and effort and increases stress levels by depriving your gray matter of valuable glucose.

It does not make you more efficient. Moving from one thing to another takes time and your brain can only process a few things at any one time. Depressingly few of them. It is all about the energy cost to cognitive processes of attentional switching.

Your brain can give its attention to only a small number of stimuli at any one time. The fewer, the better. Miller (1956) proposed we can handle seven +/- two pieces of information at once. But the number may actually be four or even fewer (Cowan, 2001).

Given that it takes a finite time to move your attention from one task to another, you will be more efficient if you do one thing, do it well and complete it.

Multi-tasking is a term from computer science: Rather than feed one task into the central processing unit (CPU - the computer's active calculating brain part) at a time, two or more processes can be threaded at once. The CPU does one part from one job, moves to another, does this and moves back to the first. It gives the illusion of performing two things at once, but still calculates one thing at a time (albeit quite fast) and turns its attention to the next.

If the world's most powerful computers can't actually manage more than one thing at a time, what chance to we have? To be effective, we should focus on one thing and one thing only. The thing in front of you. Do that until it is done and then do the next thing. Use your triage skills (not separating into three, it derives from the French word *trier*, meaning to sift) and the Pareto principle (80/20 rule) to prioritize your tasks. Then do them in order. That is it.

Achieving this is tricky as evidenced by a whole industry of self-help books (including by me) to help you get off your butt, into gear and into effective daily action. Get those distractions away. Set your day up to not be interrupted. Your newsfeed doesn't need checking nearly as often as you think. Most emails will wait until later that day; similarly your texts, voicemails, tweets and the status updates of your friends. Set aside specific time to deal with these.

One-tasking it:
- Get rid of anything which forces you to try to multi-task. Like alerts on emails, ringing phones, the book of faces and your twitter feed.
- Review your news addiction. Do you really need to refresh the page every twenty minutes? Could you perhaps look at the news at the beginning and at the end of the day? Some patients gain great benefit and increases to their productivity from this. They go on a 'news diet' - I'll bet you didn't even know that was a thing. No news from any source for a month. Or even two. They find that while tricky at first, it frees up much time and doesn't actually negatively impact on their life at all. Some get very excited about this and proselytize.
- Partition your time carefully, do the important tasks and schedule time-aside for all other less-important stuff. Stick to it.
- If you are coping, then great - do what you like. Well done you, you clever sausage.

For the rest of us - heed the message of not trying in vain to multi-task efficiently. Try to single-task. Do it, try it out.

It will feel weird at first as with any new habit. Just like a new pair of shoes. You know you need them, so put them on and wear them daily.

Eventually this new way of working will become your new

norm and feel normal. This will free up your attentional resources to manage the stuff you do, but better. It will help others in your work-space to see your boundaries. It will help you become more aware of your boundaries, where they are, just who set them and will give you some control of where they need to be. Be the one who is in charge of who tweaks them, when and for why.

having a done list

Consider having a done list.

Like a 'to-do list' but better. To-do lists are full of stuff that you are needing to do. By definition, you've not done them yet and are likely to feel the pressure of the number of tasks. The volume of mine expands faster than I can cross them off. They exist as an externalizer of my memory. Rather than spending cognitive power trying to remember tasks; writing these down, or capturing them electronically is very handy.

Great. But if this thing is weighing on you that is unhelpful. Recovering from burnout means changing stuff around to make life feel easier. That is where a done list comes in. Write down what you've done today. Include small stuff at first to get you into the swing;

- got up.
- brushed teeth.
- got to work.
- saw a patient.
- drank some coffee.
- survived the morning.
- went for a walk.
- practiced deep breathing.
- posted a letter (ok, that's going to sounds pretty archaic as this book becomes older).

When we complete tasks, this releases dopamine. The reward chemical. Completion of tasks is good. A 'done-list' still acts as a memory externalizer as you are able to spot what is still to-do (your brain is clever that way), but it feels better to strike all this stuff off. It reminds you that you are capable of action. Lots of actions. Every day. Many people can't do these things. Some of our patients cannot even go to the bathroom without assistance. You do a lot of stuff quite successfully. Don't overlook your achievements, however small and unimportant they may seem.

identity theft

Can someone steal who you are? Would you be pleased about this? Becoming depersonalized is part of the definition of burnout. The stress and pressures of your job have taken away your sense of self or changed it for the worse.

You are the sum of your parts:

> *"Everything that has passed before had to do so for you to become who you are now. It was all necessary."*
> (Hawker, 2015)

But when you burn out, you become depersonalized. This precious 'you' feels like it has gone. If you then cannot practise medicine as a consequence you are going to feel that loss too. You may question your very identity if you have the doctor part taken away as it forms such a massive part of each of our lives and who we perceive ourselves to be.

For us to be good at what we do, we invest a lot of time, mental effort and countless precious hours of our lives trying to help others the best way that we know how. Inevitably this leaves a mark, a huge chunk of our sense of self becomes invested in this. Literally our brains have become configured to be physicians. When pathways fire together, they wire together, they strengthen and reinforce. These neural pathways actually physically grow when we use them more.

London cabbies increase the size their hippocampus during their acquisition of 'The Knowledge' and during the years after (Maguire, Woollett and Spiers, 2006).

There is no reason to believe that similar changes don't happen in the brains of medics. We study for just as long. And longer. We spend just as much time training and working for professional qualifications. For decades.

So if you suddenly stop doing that, or find your capacity has diminished for whatever reason, you are going to notice a bit of a hole.

Working out what to do with that will be a challenge. And will be different for each of us. So when you cut back on the hours put in at work or otherwise disconnect and step off the crazy hamster wheel, you will need to fill some hours with non work-related activities.

Whether you fill the attentional gaps with fluff (crosswords, wine, an affair, psychoactive chemicals) or something more constructive is up to you. To do so with some attention and careful thought seems smart.

It is all too easy to hit the mental snooze button and this can readily turn into an unhelpful habit which then can take a bit of deconstructing, realigning and reconfiguring the best way to aim your considerable brain with its capacity for higher and complex mental functioning.

These skills after all are what we've worked at for years to make you a doc.

What makes a doc?
- *Knowledge, lots of facts.*
- *Knowing how the brain works, the body, the physiology, the complex interplay of us as humans in sickness and in health.*
- *Awareness of how it all fits together in the wider health community. The relevance of modern medicine advances.*
- *Medicines and healthcare interventions.*
- *Statistics and probabilities.*
- *Healthcare behavior and the patient in their social setting.*
- *Society's expectations and the complex way we behave towards each other.*
- *How to help people motivate and generate their own coping strategies to become well, to stay well and to best cope with what may come in the future.*

All this and much more. We manage all this because of and in spite of being people with lives, social lives, leisure pursuits and families. In a world where we all demand more for less, faster and faster responses to the spiraling demands, we have to be perfect. We are held to higher and higher standards from ourselves, society and our patients.

But we remain fallible and human underneath. We sometimes forget this.

priorities

Your number one priority is to look after number one.

This axiom of better self-care applies whether you are Mr Nasty or Mr Nice guy (or gal obviously):

- Some people are selfish; they should look after number one. As, for them they are the most important person in the universe and it stands to reason that their needs come first.
- Some people care deeply about others, but they too should look after number one. To adequately care for others and to dedicate each waking moment to looking after someone else or making the world a better place to live in, you are going to need to be functioning well, with enough physical and emotional resources for the job. Well fed, not tired and inadequately rested. This is because you cannot give from an empty cup.

Lots of people in the so-called caring professions spend their lives looking after others; their families, their colleagues, their friends, their children and their patients. Next on the priority list is them. But the list is so long and so demanding that there isn't often any time left at the end of the day for self care.

The trouble with this strategy is that it won't work forever. You will break. Like a car which doesn't get serviced. Eventually a bit is going to fall off / seize up / or otherwise go kaput.

So, your number one priority is you.

Gandhi once remarked that as tomorrow was a going to be a really busy day, he would spend twice as long in his morning meditation. He had a good point.

are you depressed?

Depression affects a lot of people (Kessler and Bromet, 2013; NIMH, 2014):
- It has a prevalence of 9% (29% in physicians).
- It has an annual incidence of 6.7% in the general population.
- It has a lifetime incidence in the general population of 4% for males and 9% for females (13% in male medics and 20% for female medics).

Medics consistently outperform the general population in study after study. We seem to have an occupational bonus which summates on the background risk, as inconveniently we also happen to be people (Frank and Dingle, 1999; Goldman, Shah and Bernstein, 2015; Mata et al, 2015; Schwenk, 2015).

The completed suicide rate among physicians (40 per 100,000) is double that of the general population (Miller et al, 2000; Schernhammer and Colditz, 2004; Petersen and Burnett, 2008). Not very good news.

In case you are rusty, the ICD-10 definition of depression is: **a mood disorder with persistent sadness or low mood and/ or loss of interests or pleasure, fatigue or low energy. At least one of these features most days, most of the time and for at least two weeks** (ICD-10, 2015).

The biological features of depression are thought to be treatable and to respond to either or both a talking therapy approach or anti-depressant medication. If you have these features, then consider fixing something. Sometimes talking to a colleague, loved one or professional will do the trick.

Cognitive behavioral therapy (CBT) works particularly well for doctors who are solution oriented, articulate, motivated and can handle with ease the small amount of focused homework after each session (Guille et al, 2015).

Perhaps a little more self-care and adequate sleep will help. If not - then consider taking medication which alters your neurochemistry - no, not those ones. I'm talking about SSRIs or TCADs. Basically if the other actions don't work then see your doctor and talk through the pros and cons of prescription medication.

do you become anxious?

Anxiety is more common than you might think. Both in terms of the general population (which of course we all belong to, admit it or not) and in doctors (Andrew, 2006; Cole and Carlin, 2009; Bianchi et al, 2015; Mata et al, 2015).

It can manifest in many ways. I have a friend who uses bulimic purging as a way of controlling stuff in her life. She is a doctor and finds that this gives a sense of control. She can see that there are better and more healthy coping strategies, but finds this provides a release that nothing else does.

I'm not suggesting that for you. In fact I suggest the opposite. But having tough days and fielding impossible demands is a way of life for many. Some of us turn to booze, some hide in drugs. Gambling and sex addictions can snare us likewise. For others, the lure of the illicit affair or casual liaison is an irresistible let-off for perceived pent up steam.

The pent up steam theory may be understandable, but may not be valid as it is not admissible in a court of law. In all the many years of case-law it has never been shown to have a convincing peer-reviewed evidence base.

Sometimes anxiety can manifest as avoiding of social situations. Simple social avoidance is high on the list of ways of coping with this social phobia. Not really a proper phobia, it is simply an avoidance behavior. Keeping your office door closed. Not answering calls. Leaving your email unchecked. Allowing your post to accumulate.

Discharge summaries and letters left undictated sometimes belie an underlying anxiety.

We are all perfectionists and want to do well. If we don't see the patient, don't do the visit, don't check the request; then we can't fail, right? We can't get it wrong, we can't be found to be wanting.

But we are also professionals. It forms part of your self esteem to do your job well, and rightly so. It is all tied up. It is important for us to hold our head up high and unfortunately this often involves not putting stuff off. You owe it to yourself, your patients and your colleagues to be prompt.

Anxiety is worry about something out of proportion to the actual threat. By definition it is too high. It is normal and reasonable to be cautious and indeed careful in all of your life. For you and your patients.

Defining what are reasonable and what are not reasonable risks and threats can prove to be a challenge. Sometimes the lines aren't very clear. If they are not clear and it doesn't cause a problem then so what? But if it is making you feel bad and affecting your professional performance and / or your personal life, then something has to give.

stress stuff

Stress is the perception of overwhelm.

A disparity between perceived pressure on one side and coping outlets / ability to perform the tasks on the other. Sometimes we feel stress over things that perhaps aren't *that* important when you take in the bigger picture.

Take a meta picture: Helicopter up to survey the situation from on high. Fly above your problems. From this higher up vantage point they may appear as small obstacles or stepping stones rather than impenetrable walls or unsurmountable hurdles.

Take the long view - in ten years time how much of this will really matter?

Sometimes it can be useful to remember that in the grand scheme of things you are not really vital (sorry to have to break that to you). You are a few kilograms of carbon atoms, a few gallons of water and some extra bits and bobs. You carry a genetic code for making similar copies of yourself and that is about it. Oh, and the carrying around of billions of micro-organisms in your human biome. I appreciate that it is helpful to ascribe meaning and importance to this passing on of the genes, but from the planetary perspective, it will get along fine without you. You are a but tiny relatively unimportant cog and this is a good thing. You can take time out and the world will keep turning. You can put everything on pause, step back, re-evaluate, recharge and then re-engage when everything feels better. The world will still be out there. It may not even have noticed that you had gone AWOL for a bit.

Your life may of course improve if you do nothing. But it

doesn't tend to very often. One definition of madness if keeping doing the same thing and expecting different results.

If you keep doing what you've always done, you will tend to get what you've always got.

Are you over-doing things? If so, stop and ease back. Consider your inner driving voices. Which ones are being helpful and supportive? Is there a part of your internal dialog which constantly questions your actions, tells you that you're doing it wrong, are worthless and will never amount to anything? It might be time to start ignoring that particular voice or at least turn its volume right down to the level of background noise. Keep the helpful ones - those that unlink your esteem and ego from your sense of self, your wellbeing and from your work performance.

Keep some perspective. Even in burnout this isn't the end of everything and the world as we know it. Banish those depressive, nihilistic, suicidal thoughts. Next time a voice labels you as a failure, realize it is simply a nasty bully and needs to be kicked in the gonads. I mean ignored or stood up to. Disregard the lies.

Find the silver lining. This time of self reflection and re-evaulation of goals, strategies and relationships is a great chance to reconnect with the inner and most splendid you.

Some people like to consider that you are as a pretty diamond. But covered in horse shit. For years you've been applying nail varnish to the outside to keep a thin veneer of niceness and make it look better. But the stink is all pervasive. Allow the outer layers to fall away. Stop this silly covering up. Clean up the horse shit and allow your inner diamond out. Let it shine in the bright morning sun. Glinting away. Not evidenced based, I grant you, but some people find the imagery helpful.

Or simply take time to chill out. **Don't sweat the small stuff … And it's all small stuff!!**

self-care

I get a sore throat when I'm feeling low. It can come on within hours of not looking after myself. Whether it is dehydration, self-pity or an actual manifestation of a lowered immune system is for cleverer doctors than me to pontificate. As a junior doctor and as a young(er) adult I had the throat thing a lot. This scratchy throat symptom turned up mid-night shift or if I'd neglected my sleep. I used to burn the candle at both ends. Not a good long term coping strategy I grant you, but it helped me feel that life wasn't all work and no fun.

I missed the bigger picture of looking after one's self. I'm older and wiser, well more experienced anyway, now. The harder I push myself, the more the throat hurts, even within a few hours. Rest more and it's better by the next day. Less rest and it drags on for days. I've encountered this in many of my patients too and offer it as a seaweed blowing in the wind point (occasionally accurate).

Just how do we take better care of ourselves and prevent or cure burnout? A good question and I'm glad you asked. We don't really know the best strategies for helping occupational burnout. Compassion seems to help a bit (Thakur, 2015). Basically, there is no compelling evidence on the efficacy of the different interventions (relaxation / meditation / CBT / changing work schedules). So what does all that mean?

Cochrane updated a review in 2014 and found not an awful lot. The papers weren't terribly robust in terms of control and had woolly outcomes (such as 'less stress' - whatever that may actually mean in real terms). The follow up was short (one to six months in many of the studies analyzed). The participant numbers were also small. Though this isn't really surprising in that there isn't a lot of money to be made from this (Ruotsalainen et al, 2014).

I feel this is nearsighted of big employers and that they might want increased productivity in the workforce and fewer days off sick with a happier workplace, I would have thought would be worth plowing a few millions of research money into... but what would I know.

There are a million variables in your's and everyone else's life - drinking, infections, relationships, happiness, wellbeing, increased inflammation within your atherosclerotic plaques and how well your DNA repair mechanisms fend off developing cancers. Basically, it is going to be impossible to get hard data.

So we are going to have to address woolly outcomes in a woolly subject with woolly strategies. You aren't going to be able to look this stuff up very well.

So go with your gut. Probably go with what seems to work for your patients. I would be tempted by mainstream wins like sleep, diet and exercise over homeopathy and anything that involves invisible energy alignment.

Probably do more self care. Find more time in your life to take care of someone important. You. Sandwich it into your day or plan around it. But it has to go in somewhere - or you will break. And if you are already broken, stop and mend before anything else.

Take your time:
- Time to look after yourself.
- Time to unwind.
- Time to pursue a leisure life.
- Time in nature, outdoors, for sport, with family, loved ones and friends.
- Time to enjoy good food, literature, music, art and films.
- Time to read.
- Time to write.

The mental space for all of these will come with deliberate focus. It tends not to happen if you don't actively pursue it. I find running gives me the biggest return on investment of time and effort - it feels good, makes me fitter, de-stresses me, curbs my waistline, gets me outside, lets me listen to music, doesn't cost much, energizes me, is likely to make me live longer and makes me a nicer person to be around albeit a bit smellier and more disheveled.

Carving out space in your life for you can feel all too selfish. I contest that this isn't selfish and I would go onto argue that you are selfish if you do not do this.

You owe it to your friends, family and loved ones to be the best you can be. You owe it to your patients as a professional and as a human being to be the kindest, nicest, best educated and most functional doctor you can be. Most of all, you owe it to you.

You are alive for a set number of minutes on this planet. I'm not very impressed by the alarmingly few of these that I'm likely to have left. It is up to you to make the most of your's. You don't have to of course. You can do what you like.

But it seems from those people who consider these things, that living life to the full, connecting with others, sharing experiences and savoring moments is what brings the best reward for the efforts spent in trying to have a great day (Maslow, 1943; Kübler-Ross, 1969; Sargent et al, 1977; van Dierendonck et al, 2005; Gawande, 2015; Hawker, 2015).

Tips for better self-care:
- take your lunch hour.
- take all your annual leave.
- leave work on time.
- don't be contactable outside work.
- take proper sick leave if ill (that's a biggie, really do this. No excuses).

Add to your working day:
- read a novel on your commute (I use audiobooks as I drive in).

- read it more on your lunch break.
- take some fresh air.
- go to the gym.
- listen to music.
- meet a friend.

Small steps, baby steps - start with five minutes of time-out for yourself.
- It might sound silly.
- Set the timer on your phone (so you remember to do it and so it has a defined limit once you start).
- It is the thin end of a very important wedge and allows you to learn partitioning and being in the 'off' position (not computer off, simply in sleep mode.)
- *'Listen to your body'*, I tell my patients who whinge on about their aches and pains. *'What is it telling you?'* **It is screaming at you; more rest, sleep and self-care.** But you've got stuff to do… Your body doesn't know about this stuff. It doesn't care. All it knows is that it is broken, breaking or at imminent risk of breaking and to fix itself it needs you to rest and fuel better. Sleep and rest. It will tell you when it is ready.

In the old days we used to confine people to bed rest for weeks and this worked for nearly everything (venous thromboembolisms notwithstanding). We now have other stuff which helps just as much and have forgotten that they *still* need the rest. In our attempts to have zero patients with PEs and VTEs we get people up on the day of their operations.

We get people back to work to stop them indulging their sick-role. This is good for preventing some malingerers (though in my opinion not many and not nearly enough - I'm sure you feel the same). But it is at the expense of people with real unwellness which needs real time off, real rest and real sleep. For days, weeks and sometimes even months. It may well be that a stitch in time saves nine and while I have no good evidence for this - it seems to work in my own life.

So listen. Stop when your body tells you and don't get up until you are ready. This will, I firmly believe, help you be more functional overall. It will get you back to health faster and help you to work better once you are there.

consultation antecedents

We bring stuff (read: *baggage*), along with us to each clinical and professional encounter (read: *everyone we meet at work*).

Few of us travel light. The stuff that has gone on in our lives before and the stuff which is going on in our lives in the background permeates our everyday interactions. When you are burning out, the professional front becomes progressively harder to maintain. When it slips we need to take action. The challenge here is in the early recognizing.

Before a consultation there is stuff that happens. This affects and colors both the interaction and the outcome. Being more aware of this stuff can allow the clinician to steer and facilitate a more effective consultation.

These principles were outlined by Pendelton et al (2003). Among the things the patient brings are their ideas, concerns and expectations. These in turn are colored by their prior knowledge. They are affected by the newspaper articles they've seen, television shows, things their family have told them, doctor-google, the wikipedia article and so on.

What the doctor brings is a pre-judgment on the case. A working diagnosis and plan from the get-go. We bring the knowledge we are sure of, the gaps, the previous cases we remember (a case study being of course the least valid form of evidence but often the best shared and recalled). We bring previous experience but also our personal life. We bring background thoughts of our relationship issues, our aches and pains, we bring the state of our bowels and if our tummies are well fed. Whether our children are ill, if there is a tax bill due and so on. These will all color our judgment, mood and the interaction with the patient and probably also the outcome.

To deny these affects is naive. You may consult a lot better than I, but these resonate with me. The trick is to be aware of them and the potential biases and effects they may provide and then to work with what you've got.

The higher your stress levels, the more burned out you are, the fewer mental resources you've got for spotting these and managing them. And probably also the worse the impact is.

after seeing patients

After the dust has settled on the consultation or interaction, you and the patient go your separate ways. The party is over and the parties have parted and departed. Now there are the left-overs that need clearing up. Mental processes and lingering thoughts. You need a reset before the next patient in order to maintain sanity and to bring your best untainted self to the next one. There was a good book on this: *Housekeeping - the good housekeeping guide*.

It should have been called that. Maybe. Actually titled 'The Inner Consultation: How to Develop an Effective and Intuitive Consulting Style' and penned by Roger Neighbour (1987).

This approach is applicable across specialties. He advocated performing a mental re-set after each patient. Clearing the decks of psychological clutter and thought debris between patients is something that helps the wheels of cognition run more smoothly.

We remind our trainees that the last patient of the day is as deserving as the first patient. There are doctor factors which affect each consultation and each patient interaction. And indeed each professional conversation.

There is also the so-called 'lunch effect' first published by Tversky and Kahneman in Science (1974) where they showed parole hearings scheduled before lunch were significantly less likely to be granted than just after. This mental switching off when we are hungry extends to other internal mental processes (Danzigera et al, 2011). These internal biases may well be something we are blind to (like the noise of a refrigerator until it stops working).

Keeping a sense of self-awareness as we progress through our days helps us notice when we are keeping emotional clutter in our heads. It is all too easy to do.

Having a mental clear out between each patient is a sensible idea. You may of course already do this to a super-high standard. I suspect I don't manage this nearly as well as I claim at my annual appraisal. If you need a steer on how to feel better between patients, the solution is as straightforward and easy to apply as taking a deep breath, relaxing the excess tension from your muscles (having your tongue not pressed hard against your palate and unclenching the fists is a good start), putting a smile on your face and correcting your posture. This is all you need for the moment.

With a little practice, that can be done in the blink of an eye. Or three luxuriant seconds. Whichever works best for you.

How do we start recovering from burnout? Doing nothing probably won't be very effective. A poor choice. It doesn't tend to go away on its own. It may get worse. And if it does, you may well not be very well placed to notice.

Addressing the underlying issues is key. There will be some you can change and some you can't. The ones you cannot change now, you may be able to in future and you may be able to find satisfactory work-around solutions to carry you forward from here. Action sooner rather than later works for most things in life and burnout would seem to be one of these.

The recovery is not something to do one weekend. Like dieting and improving your waistline, you will get the best long term results if you have consistent, carefully directed actions. Ones which you are able to continue for the rest of your life, which include building in steps for future resilience and alertness to warning signs in the future.

Burnout requires time and space to go away. Rest, recuperation and time to fully recover are part of this. Weeks and months may be involved. Outside assistance is very very helpful. Difficult to ask for and difficult to accept (you are a physician after all, and asking for help and accepting fallibility is beaten out of us in medical school and usually embraced internally as the years tick by).

- Consider keeping a stress diary.
- Try recording a worry diary.
- Set aside a specific 'worry time of day', allocate five to ten minutes. Vow not to spend any of your other all too valuable seconds on worries. Simply note them down when they occur and save them up for 18h00 each day when you allow yourself a few minutes dedicated fretting time. When the time is up - move on. Tomorrow's worry session will come along soon enough.

alcohol

Alcohol is frequently used and misused by doctors and patients alike. Both for fun and as a coping strategy.

Just because it is widespread, this doesn't make it a good idea. Don't forget your basic physiology. It takes time to process the ethanol and until it has left your system there is frontal lobe suppression (which feels nice but impairs effective sleep).

When I went to medical school there was a drinking culture. The cool kids drank. The coolest parties with the highest perceived social currency were full of liquor. The funniest antics of my peers were fueled by ethanol. These were condoned by the university in that they facilitated the running of the bar and a blind eye was turned to all but the most extreme acts.

> *"I spent a lot of money on booze, birds and fast cars. The rest I just squandered."*
>
> (George Best, Footballer)

It was regarded as letting off steam and a natural way for budding doctors to behave. After all what is wrong with a little high spirits and high jinks? Once we qualified we would of course become pillars of society...

This didn't happen all at once, what changed was the alcohol became consumed from more expensive bottles and usually over many courses of dinner. There was as the years went by a little less late night dancing. But still the volatile liquid flowed.

Hospital mess parties took the place of medical school fresher's week and here much debauchery took place and was almost encouraged. It was after all grand tradition. Generations before had done this and we are all for supporting the earliest traditions of our noble profession, are we not?

As the years ticked by and we settled into our respective specialties, much of the damage had already been done. Many doctors remained in debt with strings of unsuccessful relationships and divorces. The increasing pressures of professional exams and young families pushed drinking to fewer and fewer occasions, but somehow we still behaved like we were making up for lost time and there were simply harder binges on those nights.

Many others simply settled into a pattern of a bottle of wine after work each night - between two of you, obviously (more would be greedy). But starting off with a couple of cheeky beers or a restorative gin and tonic didn't really count, did it?

Drinking more than about 14 units a week is probably not healthy for anyone. This relatively arbitrary number doesn't match the health benefits of halving that. It's just that successive governments in the UK haven't had the political chutzpah to come out and say it.

This would be deeply unpopular and thus has been skirted and dodged by politicians who are famous for being heavy on the rhetoric while light on actions and for heavy and regular alcohol consumption (usually quite expensive, good vintages at the expense of the public purse too - but that is a discussion for another day).

In the public eye, the only people who drink more than politicians are doctors. The commonest cases in front of our professional boards are alcohol related misdemeanors (driving DUIs and being intoxicated at work).

__The definition of an alcoholic is someone who drinks more than their doctor.__

- I'm hopeful the tide is turning.
- In the UK it is ten years since a smoking ban in public came

through. In its wake smoking has shifted from being socially ok, to socially not ok. Doctors who smoke are now rare.

Drinking is slowly going the same way. It used to be ok to be a bit drunk and drive (not legally - I mean socially, people turned a blind eye to this). It is now not really ok to admit you've got a drink driving ban. While heavy drinking is expected of doctors - the acceptability is dropping. No longer is it ok for a doctor to be inebriated in public. Public opinion is driven by the popular press who sensationalize when doctors misbehave. It's not anything to do with work but they expect us to hold higher standards than other members of society. While you can debate the merits of either stance, for burnout: if you drink, the writing is on the wall.

Consider cutting it, seeking help or otherwise modifying it to include alcohol free days each week. Do not consume too much in one session. Or if you do - do it with awareness and not merely as a mental, social or psychological crutch when there are other things that could do this better and in a more healthy manner.

memory function

Your frontal lobes are awesome. They represent a pinnacle of evolution up and away from the animals. They think, fantasize, organize, plan, sift your memories, problem solve and sort out your mental hangups. Your brain acts as your personal psychiatrist. It will psychoanalyze and iron out your mental wrinkles. And the coolest part of all is this happens while you are asleep.

If you sedate your brain (sleeping tablets, alcohol and even SSRIs) they don't do this nearly as well. You need your eight hours of beauty sleep for them to work this magic in the background. For it to fire on all cylinders and power away your problems while you are blissfully unaware, you need to give yourself the physical and temporal space to allow for this arcane action.

If you do not get adequate rest, your cognitive function declines (Walker et al, 2003; Stickgold and Matthew, 2007; Ferrie et al, 2011).

Sleep well and the organizing power of the mind will do all of this splendid stuff in the background. No effort required on your part. This represents a massive return on investment. Prioritize this in your life and good things will follow as surely as day follows night.

drugs

Prescription drugs and street drugs.

"I used to have a drug problem, now I make enough money."
(David Lee Roth, Rock star)

Drug use is more common in our profession than many like to admit. It can start innocuously and tends to slide. It is a good barometer for other stuff going wrong. A good surrogate marker for needing to stop, take stock and correct things (DesRoches et al, 2010).

Obviously there are good and carefully clear guidelines on this and on keeping and staying well. All that probity stuff. We should all seek help from our personal physicians when we are in need.

But the reluctance to do this is rife and perhaps understandable (DuPont et al, 2009). Whether this is morally excusable is not for me to say and that discussion is well beyond the scope of this book. You may recognize yourself or your colleague here. Reading this book (or one of many other excellent ones available) and working through the exercises can provide a lifeline and help one become more well again.

There is hope. But only once the problem is recognized, acknowledged and acted upon. I'm not talking the woo woo of 'the twelve steps' (really helpful for some people, but heavy on the god and has very little in terms of a proper evidence base). I'm talking about the sheer practicalities of spotting that things are a bit awry or at very least need some reflecting on as to whether they could be better.

Plus the illegalities of drugs; prescription and otherwise could land you in hot water and the press do love to tell the stories. Your medical board too take a dim view of this.

Take stock. Take a deep breath and either address this without delay or seek help. Probably also do this today.

do you have Starbucks shares?

Caffeine is the world's most commonly used psychotropic drug. So common indeed to be nearly universal.

Caffeine isn't all bad. It can even make you function a bit better. But why?

It increases mental alertness by sensitizing our body tissues to circulating catecholamines. In the context of burnout, the question is - are you using it to mask a lack of mental alertness that we should perhaps be paying attention to?

The commonest underlying issue is not enough sleep. Not getting enough sleep on a school night is not really ok.

Sometimes our young babies scream, our neighbors row, our children vomit and we have little choice over this. Sometimes we book holidays which take it to the wire and we fly back at the last minute. Sometimes we stay out late drinking and partying - that's less ok.

Occasionally you will bump up against life's little hiccups and that is fair enough. You need your rest and recuperation as much as the next doctor. But are you doing this out of a persistent and driving pressure to find escape and solace from a high pressured job that you're not coping with nearly as well you would like?

If this is the case, then early bed and a yoga class will give you more mental staying power than a disco and three espressos.

If you drink caffeine, you may be aware that its effects can last long into the night as you lie in bed, exhausted with the palpitations and tachycardia from increased stroke volume induced by the caffeine, *then* you don't sleep well, *then* the next day you are shattered, *then* you drink more caffeine to counter this, *then* you lie awake and so on.

If you aren't sure if you need to do something about caffeine: go full zero and and full decaffeinated for three whole weeks. Yes, even at the weekends. If your life gets better; then it was the caffeine. Reintroduce it slowly and find your tolerance level. Some people use midday as their cut off for their last caffeinated drink of the day.

Try that out.

smoking

Do you smoke? You know it is bad for you. But do you do it anyway?

Is this to be sociable? Is it just with alcohol on a night out? Beer group pressure. Is it flipping the bird to societal norms and to establish that you can make your own decisions? Is it to relieve stress?

It could be a surrogate marker for stress. You might of course have thought it out well and examined the arguments and made a reasonable decision which works for you and your life. If so, great. Good luck to you. I really don't care what you do in your private life. As long as you are happy.

If you aren't happy and things are pressing upon you, then consider addressing this one.

It can be a *gateway habit*.

A gateway habit, or keystone habit is one which, if tackled and progress made, seems to exert an effect on the rest of people's lives in that everything else gets better, the person feels better, does more and improves multiple areas of their life as a bit of serendipity, all as a happy side effect of initially changing just that one area.

what is your mental snooze alarm?

- Coffee.
- Gambling.
- Sex addiction.
- Drugs.
- Food.
- Alcohol.
- Parties.
- Affairs.

Anything that basically you know just isn't very healthy. The sort of thing your grandmother would have denounced. Many of us engage in distraction stuff. Some of it relatively innocuous like reading the newspaper, checking the book of faces, doing sudokus or crosswords, staring out of the window, or working our way through box sets. But much of this mental fluff and flimflam is just that. Not very constructive. Are there more effective ways to be spending your downtime? Are any of them potentially harmful to you, your relationships or work reputation?

You are a doctor. You've got the letters. You know your stuff. You are thus running out of excuses.

You may want to consider looking at:
- *SMART* goals.
- *SWOT* analysis.

(**s**pecific, **m**easurable, **a**chievable, **r**ealistic and **t**ime defined)
(**s**trengths, **w**eaknesses, **o**pportunities and **t**hreats of a change)

These are basic rubrics and can be used as a starting point. No right or wrongs with these, but we need to start somewhere.

Becoming more ascetic can be a trigger to greater things. Even if you don't really fancy it. Gateway habits are good like that. But if the moral high road doesn't appeal that much you could try another way of calming your inner self. Some people do well from building pauses into their life.

- Set a reminder alarm(s) on your phone or computer (perhaps once an hour).
- Build many of these.
- Five minutes may be more than adequate each time. Stop what you are doing and simply notice stuff. Take a deep breath and notice your surroundings. Notice any thoughts and feelings. Try not to react or judge them. Simply allow them to be.
- Slow down and savor each moment.

It doesn't take long, is free and can provide a sort of mental reset. Worth a try. If you are too busy to do this, it's probably even more important to try it! One of the major monotheistic religions exhorts their devotees to pray several times a day. To outsiders this seems a bit excessive. For the followers, this is simply what they do and they don't question it. From a burnout point of view this sounds like an excellent strategy.

The benefits (apart from the metaphysical ones) are in regular breaks. No choice. Just do. Ritual and quietness. Reconnecting with what is important to you. Contemplation of sacred teachings. We too can take regular timed breaks. We will have to be proactive and lever them in. But once they are there, they could start to make a significant helpful impact and you may start to relish them, treasure them and eagerly anticipate the next one.

Perhaps try it for a month and if it isn't helping significantly (your estimation, not anyone else's), then don't do them. Do whatever else is emerging as what you need in your life in your own personal set of circumstances.

procrastination

Putting stuff off is a pretty reliable indicator that you are avoiding it. Stuff too hard, too unpleasant or with things involving personal confrontation can be the cause.

> **'Don't forget - the patient is the one with the disease.'**

No matter how awkward the encounter, how unpleasant they are or how mean we have to be to give the news; at the end of the day we don't have the condition and can go and have supper with our family. They will still have whatever it is.

> *'They say if the most important thing you have to do today is eat a live frog, that it doesn't pay to stare at it for too long.'*

Popular self-help books oft mis-attribute this witticism to Mark Twain. The actual origin is Monsieur Nicolas Chamfort. A French aristocrat who in his support of the French revolution in 1790 quoted in an essay:

"M. de Lassay, a very indulgent man, but with a great knowledge of society, said that we should swallow a toad every morning, in order to fortify ourselves against the disgust of the rest of the day, when we have to spend it in society."

This has morphed into the popular concept of eating a frog as a metaphor for addressing our biggest and ugliest challenge head on. As the first task of the day. This approach to procrastination carries plenty of merit.

So the recommended approach to overcoming procrastination is don't sweat it. Crack on with whatever it was that you are avoiding. Eat that ugly toad (Sainte-Beuve, 1851).

Dr Phil Harley

workbook

This is practical stuff to try. Some of it will work for you. Some might not work just at present. That is ok. Come back to it. Re-read the book when it seems it will be more helpful for you. Some other stuff may speak to you louder at that point.

There is a lifewheel. This is a stock taking exercise which uses a visual to prompt mental actions about potential areas to take action.

A brief look at goals follows. How to set them according to some authorities and some tips.

Next we have healthy habits. I'm sure your's are great. But just in case some inspiration would be helpful, we have something to consider.

Progressive relaxation helps many of my patients and colleagues. Mindfulness can be super-helpful when you're in the right frame of mind. And can even be of value even when you're not. We have two exercises of each that work very well, are cheap and no one is going to think you are weird. Probably.

life wheel

Taking stock

This is a simple exercise and can help you look at your current situation. I find this useful with some patients to help them take a step outside the problem and look at things from a different angle. There are hundreds of variants. I typically bring up a picture in a browser window from my favorite search engine. Then print that live with the patient. We then score areas of their life from terrible (zero) to excellent (ten).

This is the unfettered wheel.

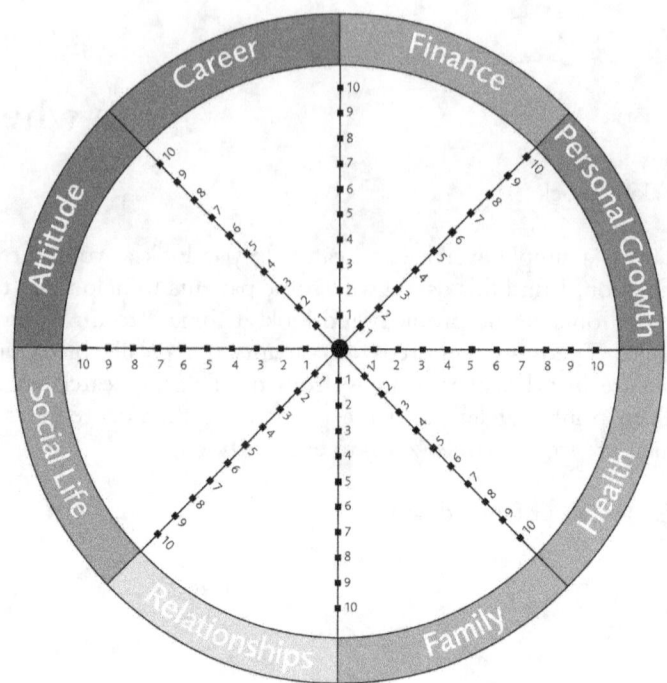

This is a typical set of answers. This provides a nice visual image and allows them to share any thoughts or insights that strike them. I ask them to make a few plans that we can review at our next session to address the areas of biggest need or that they feel will have the biggest positive impact.

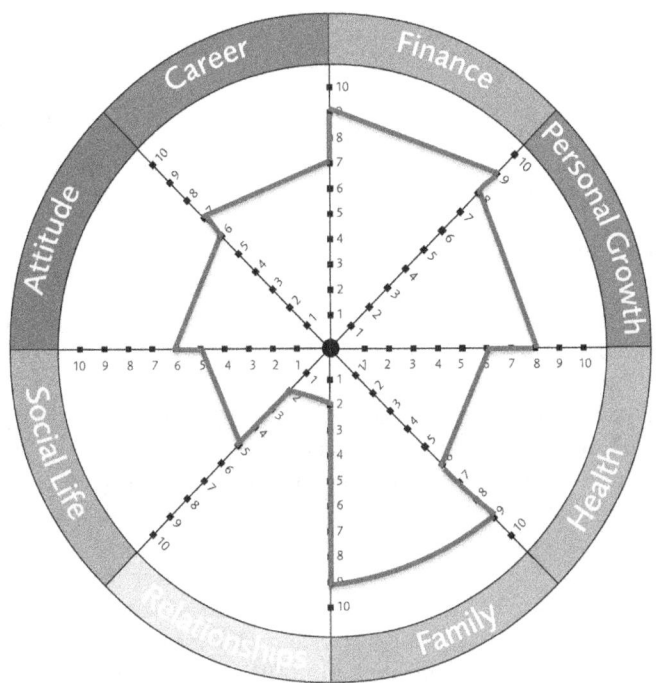

It works for doctors too. Try it. As with so many of these things, simply visualizing it in your mind isn't nearly as good as using a real pen on a real piece of paper.

goals

Make them smart.

What do you *really* want?

Are they aligned to your deeper values / religious principles / guiding beliefs?

If you already set great goals, then well, err, great. If your goals don't get you up early in the morning and keep you up late at night burning with joy, enthusiasm and a deep sense of heartfelt meaning and purpose then you might want to try setting them a little differently.

Smart goals have been around for decades now and are a nicely packaged way of defining a few characteristics which seem to be helpful in those goals that motivate people and actually get done. Loosely defined goals tend not to get completed and unrealistic goals tend to remain as daydreams.

Try using the 'smart' criteria. This acronym stands for simple, measurable, achievable, realistic and time defined.

An example of a non-smart goal could be: I want to be thinner. But: How thin? How will I know if I've achieved that? Is it in my capacity? By when? All a bit too vague.

An example of a smart goal variant could be: I want to be a size ten by Christmas. Ten = specific and measurable (I will or will not fit into *that* little black number). Achievable (I'm a twelve on a really good day now). It's realistic in that one pound a week for the next four months should get me pretty close and I've shed some of my curvy bits at that rate before. It is time defined. There is the Christmas office party and that is on the 22nd December this year.

If you write the goals down on a bit of paper with a pen, this seems to help. There is also some evidence that making a public commitment and carrying it around you in your pocket helps (Burn and Oskamp, 1986).

Checking in with your goals at intervals (try daily or once a week) reminds you what you are trying to achieve. Breaking down the goal to smaller achievable sub-goals and further individual daily tasks seems to help too (Lyubomirsky and Layous, 2013).

What no-one tells you is that if you find on your life's journey that your goals shift or your motivation wanes, then you get to re-write them or adjust them on they fly.

Why not? They are yours after all. But some of my patients it seems are too afraid to tinker once they've put them down onto paper. They feel that the goals are written in stone and then beat themselves up for not achieving what they set out to do. I say to that - 'you silly goose. They are there to help you'. I would argue that if you aren't tinkering and adjusting as you go along that you probably aren't giving them the daily attention and focus they deserve.

You may have heard that people who write their goals earn ten times those who don't. This may be true, but this urban legend research never happened.

From Harvard official website:

It has been determined that no "goals study" of the Class of 1953 actually occurred. In recent years, we have received a number of requests for information on a reported study based on a survey administered to the Class of 1953 in their senior year and a follow-up study conducted ten years later. This study has been described as how one's goals at graduation related to success and annual incomes achieved during the period.

Sadly it was all fictitious. But goal writing seems to help many people anyway (Creswell et al, 2007). If you need nudges and stuff to otherwise get you moving along, you will do little harm. And in terms of time and effort expended, this would seem to fit well Pareto's 80/20.

Again - and I do appreciate I sound like a broken record; go and get a bit of paper. Write some down. Check them. Rewrite them. Put them in your pocket and look at them tomorrow. Got it? Done it yet?

Go on, I'll wait for you.

healthy habits

Habits are vital. They are important and breathe a vitality into our day by freeing up mental energy for more interesting and novel stuff. Behavioral loops that our brains can execute and run on autopilot require a lot less energy than thinking about stuff. We have thousands of routines and subroutines that we use daily. Tying our shoelaces, reversing the car into a parking space, making a drink, unlocking a door, greeting a patient, examining to confirm a diagnosis. We rely heavily on routine and habit.

A heuristic is a mental shortcut that allows our brains to conserve vital energy and mental resources in order to pay attention to the finer things of life; poetry, sports results, attractive nearby people, shopping lists, daydream fantasies and other important stuff which seems a whole lot more interesting that whatever is going on in front of you in the here and now.

When you run the routines of habit you get to do stuff without paying it much attention. World class athletes get to do their thing and impress everyone else. The same with musicians. If we allow these routines and habits to run without examining them you are likely to keep getting the same results. This is great when things are going well and you are at the top of your game. Not quite so good when things have gone a little awry or when you've inadvertently steered a little off course.

If you keep doing what you've always done, you'll keep getting the same results.

One definition of stupid optimism is doing the same thing and hoping for different results. If you've got results in your life that are not ideal, such as stress and overwhelm and you keep running the same routines and habits, not much is likely to change in the near future. The universe isn't really set up that way.

The fascinating thing about habits is that you can change any one of them. It takes a bit of conscious effort but can be done. You can learn to take a different route to work, you can learn new ways of breaking bad news, you can learn to brush your teeth with your other hand. Whatever you want, it can be done with enough effort.

Changing habits will take a conscious decision, a little willpower, then daily efforts and is likely to feel pretty uncomfortable at first, just like the proverbial new shoes. But with daily use, they become more comfortable. Early on in the change process, if you stop paying attention you are liable to slip back into your old habit. Just like a stream running down a mountain, it will take the path of least resistance and less mental effort.

It will serve you well to deliberately create a set of healthy habits. You get to choose yours. The sort of ones that have helped many of my patients (and me) include:

- Taking the stairs, never the escalator or elevator.
- Not having second helpings.
- Counting to ten before responding angrily to a provocation.
- Whenever you notice, sit up straight.
- Smile when you answer the phone.
- Walking the long way round each time (free exercise, cheaper than the gym).
- Avoiding eating between meals.
- When the alarm rings, swing your legs out of bed without hitting snooze.
- Prepare tomorrow's lunch the day before.
- Not checking for messages or texting during the working morning.
- Scanning and acting on all paperwork that day. Ok, I'll be honest, this one I've never achieved but it is next on my hit list. I promise…

Creative writing, reflective writing, problem lists. It is all supposed to be helpful. This isn't news, so why don't we do it?

Writing stuff down can seem rather daunting at first.

There are no rules. That is also a bit scary. But it can be effective (Creswell et al, 2007). All you do is simply write.

Throw it away if it makes you feel better after. You can even start with:

I am writing. I am awake, the pen is moving. I feel like an idiot. What kind of idiot transcribes their inner monologue, I'm so stressed, I'm tired. This is stupid. Oh look, a butterfly…

You may also like to consider 'random acts of kindness'.

Your work involves being nice and helping people. But it ties you up inexorably with what you do. This isn't always a good thing as accountability is everywhere as we've already noted.

But there is joy to be found in helping someone else, maybe even outside work - doing this in a covert manner is well recognized to bring about an abundance of joy. It sounds a bit far fetched I grant you, until you try it.

If you'd like some inspiration, the philanthropic website to start with is www.randomactsofkindness.org

Burnout is scary. It feels terrible. Addressing it can seem an insurmountable task. A huge challenge and at a time when you've got the least mental resources to bring to the party. But that is ok. It will get better. Take a deep breath. Sit up straight. Ease some tension from some of your muscles. Maybe try out a small smile (we don't want to go overboard here). Most of all DON'T PANIC.

I promise it all gets easier. Like those new shoes again. New habits really do get better performed, while feeling easier to do and will become autopilot sequences. It is human nature and the way the brain works. It loves to build heuristics, which are simple pathways which use less glucose. You will wire up differently.

Neurones that fire together, wire together (Maguire, Woollett and Spiers, 2006). And your neurotransmiters will adapt and assist. They can't help it. This neuroplasticity is hardwired into your brain.

And if part of your stress and you being in a bit of a funk is down to an unhelpful balance of neurotransmitters at the moment, do stuff to change the balance.

Give your brain some different things to do and focus on and it may start to work better then you expected or hoped. The science supports this (Lyubomirsky and Layous, 2013).

Try these:
The best **first step**: smile.
Step **two**: sit and stand up straight.
Step **three**: lean forward, though not too much (that would look silly) when you talk to people.

Step **four**: get better sleep (use the tips in the 'sleep' chapter earlier).
Step **five**: get more exercise.
Step **six**: eat more wholesome helpful foods and drink.

Step **seven**: relaxation techniques.
Step **eight**: re-jig the priorities in your working day.
Step **nine**: sharpen your saw. Do stuff outside. Stuff that rekindles your fire. Loved ones, films, the joy of a good book, cooking new stuff from recipes, long walks in nature, time with your children, train for a marathon, join a prayer group, take piano lessons, I don't care - anything that works for you.

progressive relaxation

I know you're a doctor. I don't want to tell you stuff you already know, but some of us don't cover relaxation techniques in our training and haven't come across anything like progressive relaxation.

This isn't rocket science. Nothing complex. If you know about it, then skip this section.

If you've not come across this before, then try it out. It's experiential. In that picturing how it feels is not going to be anywhere as good as actually doing it. The first technique of progressive relaxation takes a full five minutes and is best practiced the first few times before drifting off to sleep. The second takes fewer than thirty seconds and can even be done at a work desk.

Technique one: Progressive muscle relaxation

Does what it says on the tin. Lie down. Tense and relax all your muscles. It leaves you feeling calm, centered (whatever that means) and feel better able to face the world.

Are you lying comfortably? Shoes off, door locked, phone off? That sort of thing. Sitting can be ok too.

Scrunch your face up. Nice and tight. Feel the power in your facial muscles of expression. Orbicularis occuli, masseter, levator labii, procerus and corrugator supercilii. Hold this tension for a second or two. Just enough to notice how tight it all feels, then let it all go. Nice and relaxed and feel the contrast. Your afferent feedback will tell you how lovely and relaxed this now feels.

Next, tense your shoulders. Some people actually move them. If you simply contract in place (isometric contractions) then you will not move around too much during this. That is probably better but does take a little practice if all this is a bit new to you. With the tension in your shoulders and up the back of your neck (don't forget to include all the bunched up muscles at your occiput) all nice and tight, then again; let it all go. Feel it flow away. Maybe down your fingers and out.

Tense all the muscles down both arms. You can clench your fists and feel your upper limbs like iron. Then let it all flow away. Some people visualize here the tension going like a color or a liquid flowing away from them and vanishing. It doesn't matter how you do it - but make it work for you. I use a vivid purple which fades through deeper shades as it leaves.

Next feel the tension across your chest and upper back. Tighten and let it all go. Pay attention to the common areas of tightness across your medial trapezius and rhomboids (between your shoulder blades if anatomy classes were a little while ago).

Your lower back and abdomen are next. Use the muscles to fool the feedback loops into extra relaxing and break the reflex arc which gives so many of us non-needed muscle tension. Tighten up your lower back and all the way across your belly. Engage your transversus, your obliques and the recti (they are in there somewhere, I promise). Let all the tension flow away.

Next up; your buttocks, hips and groin. Tense up and let it all go.

Your lower limbs next. Drain all the tension left from your upper body - and there won't be much of it left by now - into your legs. Allow it to collect as you tense. And then send it away. Give it a mental push. Feel the contrast of your bunched and tense feet against what is left as all the tenseness is gone.

Then simply lie there for a few seconds. Thirty to sixty seconds of quiet, slow, long, languid, enjoyable breaths. Simply allow yourself to be in the moment. No thoughts. No urgency.

Then come back to the real world when you are ready. Shoes

back on, blinds up, phone back on and so on. Repeat as often as needed. You may find some benefit from performing this daily.

Technique two: Ten steps to rapidly de-tension

A neologism Orwell would have been proud of. Rapidly relax sounds like an oxymoron. But my friend, 'tis effective and improves with practice.

Ten actions. All associated with a slow breath.

One: *breathe in slowly. Imagine the tension draining from your scalp and down the back of your neck and off away once if reaches your lower back. Breathe out long.*

Two: *again a slow in-breath. Unclench your teeth and take the tension from your cheeks and temples (masseter and temporalis if you want specifics). Long slow breath out.*

Three: *The slow breathing continues, slow it down each time. Take all the tension from your forehead and around the eyes, allow them to close if you like. Frontalis and orbicularis occuli - actually I'm not going to keep naming them, you get the idea. Slowwwww breath out again.*

Four: *With each breath in, once you get maximal inspiration, hold it for a few seconds. The same with the breath out. Hold it once your have full expiration. This can really help slow your breathing rate. Your pulse will follow and the 'as-if' principle of psychology will generate calm relaxed feelings on the inside. Really. It really does this. Where were we? Just done the eyes. Around the mouth now. Relax all those tension lines and allow your tongue to fall away from the roof of the mouth where so many of us keep it pressed.*

Five: *Relax the front of your neck. Feel the worries of the moment seep away. Let them go.*

Six: *Relax the big tense muscles at the back of your neck. Allow them to* *soften and let the pressures of whatever is going on at the moment become more distant. Just for now.*

Seven: *Your shoulders in turn will be eased and softened as the day fades to be less important. Just for these few precious seconds.*

Eight: *Feel any pressures run down your arms and out of your fingers as tension in your upper limbs fades. Unclench those fists, they aren't helping anybody.*

Nine: *Take the pressure from between your shoulder blades, allow your chest to move more freely and let the tension flow from your torso.*

Ten: *Relax in one big colorful, happy imagination, let go all the tension in your lower back and all the way down. Let it all go. Then open your eyes when you are ready. Blink, smile and you are ready to face the world once more.*

mindfulness exercises

Exercise one: *sit in a chair and simply notice everything. Immerse yourself in the sensory experience. Visual, auditory and kinesthetic.*

Allow yourself to notice what you can see in the center of your vision. Notice colors, shapes and edges. Notice shadows and contrasts. Allow your focus to then drift outwards. Without moving your head. Allow yourself to start to notice things around the periphery. Shadows, how the colors change and how the edges swim in and out of focus. How much of the visual panorama can you become aware of at the same time?

Listen to the sounds in your head, the voices going on, the beat of your pulse. Perhaps you can hear your breathing. Start to notice the way the sounds of your clothes move with your respiration. Allow your focus to drift outwards. The sounds of traffic, the hum of the computer, the refrigerator. Sounds of distant conversation. Perhaps birdsong, music, children. Perhaps nothing other than a mild tinnitus to prompt you to change the batteries in your hearing aid.

Feel your body. Become aware of your digestion. Notice and then move on from any aches and pains. Notice your limb positions. Feel any feedback from your limbs, your toes and your fingers. Again, allow your focus to pan out. Feel the chair under you. The pressure of your butt on the cushion. Notice your feet on the floor. Feel any movement of air over your skin and so on. Immerse yourself in your senses, both inside and out. This has a great knack of quietening your mind.

Why do we neglect smell, taste and the sixth sense that someone is watching us? - I suspect this is because they don't tend to give helpful data in this exercise.

Exercise two: *sit in a comfy chair and just sit. Allow the voices in your head to go nuts and tell you all the things you should be doing more than* *any other. Give them space. They will settle down. Eventually. They are just the voices in your head, or if that sounds a bit too like something Schneider would be interested in, perhaps call them your inner monologue. Although it rarely is a monologue - gosh, there seem to be so many in there.*

Anyhow - let them all go quiet. Once they've become quiet you may start to notice you have two things emerging: A desire to do something you really want to and probably several somethings you feel that you should do.

Here's the kicker: Go and do the thing you want to. Enjoy it. Savor the moment. And THEN go and do the things you feel you should.

These two exercises are really about simply allowing yourself to become a little more aware in a detached and thus blameless way of all the stuff that is going on in your head. And also coming to realize that it is just stuff without substance, flotsam and jetsam (probably no lagan or derelict) floating around aft the transom of your mind.

Just a bunch of fleeting and not so fleeting insubstantial thoughts. There are a lot of them. You can notice them without necessarily acting on all of them. It is just information, data to help improve and guide your decision making.

If any of it bothers you or doesn't feel nice: Then allow those ones to drift away. Focus on some others. There should be plenty to choose from.

Another good thing about these exercises is that they don't take very long, are portable, free, and can be repeated as often as you feel they could be useful.

They can be done eyes closed or eyes open. Lying on your examination couch or sat in your office chair.

Usually done in private and probably best not done while driving, they can feel quite relaxing and unlike caffeine may revive you during your working day and actually help sleep when you need it a little later.

A little like meditation, mindfulness is simply a term invented to apply a label to this sort of thing. It isn't really new, religions have encouraged regular prayer which looks remarkably similar and has been helping people feel better for a few millennia now.

the end

You've reached the end. Basically:

DON'T PANIC. Take stock. Take care of yourself and ask for help.

Some more nudges which may be helpful:
- Write your ten most pressing tasks.
- 80/20 them.
- Chunk those down into manageable bite sized pieces.
- Which is the mission critical one? The biggest, fattest, juciest frog. Eating these frogs first has been espoused by everyone from Italian film directors to American presidents.

Harley priority check-ins: How's your self care project going?

Body:
- Sleep
- Exercise
- Sex drive (a surrogate marker)
- Diet quality
- Body mass index

Mind:
- Stress
- Anxiety
- Depression
- Drug use including alcohol - anything psychotropic

Spirit:
- Connect with loved ones - family circle
- Allow yourself to be in the moment
- Allow mental space

When it's terrible:
- Remember this: You are alive. This is a good thing. Many people commit suicide or work themselves to death. You've still got the edge on them.
- You have the capacity left to read this. Also good (and axiomatic).
- You have therefore got some capacity to move on.

Also remember this:
- What is gone is over. Your time is now. And your now will shape your future.
- This is not complex, but sometimes gets a bit overlooked. Focus on your here and now. Cover your basics. Like Maslow's much talked about pyramid. Get your foundations right before moving up to the next level.

Use Harley's simplified pyramid of doctor needs:
- *Eat, sleep, rest.*
- *Exercise.*
- *Play.*

Then de-clutter your work days:
- Stop stuff, say no. Move the goalposts.

Be proactive with your professional development:
- Don't neglect it, as outsiders will judge you and monitor you with this.
- It is thus smart to stay a step ahead. Even if you don't feel like fully engaging.
- Engage with your work in a proactive manner.
- Reflect on your work and engage with your professional development. Remember, it didn't happen unless you wrote it down. So write lots. You can edit it all later.

Find some goals:
- Short, medium and long.
- Achieve the short ones and feel good. This moves you forward and accelerates the process.

Find a purpose:
- You're going to have to do this one alone. I'm going to be of no practical help here.
- But a few minutes each week checking in with what drives you is likely to be time well spent.
- Follow your purpose. Being true to ourselves is fundamentally important.
- No one can steal your sense of self. Viktor Frankl documented his experiences as an Auschwitz concentration camp inmate in World War II. He described identifying a purpose in life. He immersed himself in that purpose and credits this inner drive with his survival and that of many others (Frankl, 1946).

Finally:
- Achieve Nirvana, heaven on earth and a state of enlightenment (if you get to this bit, can you email to show off / feel smug and tell me how you've managed it so I can try and copy you. Much appreciated).

about the author

Thank you for reading my book. If you enjoyed it, please leave a review online.

Dr Phil Harley enjoys running. And some other stuff. Mostly running. He lives in the Midlands, UK.

If you have any comments, thoughts, questions or feedback, please email drphil@brainsolutions.co.uk

---

More information at www.brainsolutions.co.uk
Other books by Dr Harley:

Out now:

Skinny Genes - *Weight Gain Explained & the CURE*

Desert Marathon Training - *2nd edition: Tips for Beginners*

Beginner's Guide to Running

Ultramarathon Running Injuries - *Niggles, Scrapes and Nipple Chafes*

30 Winning Weight Loss Ways - *Simple, easy, step-by-step expert diet guidance*

Doctor Secrets for Easy Weight Loss - *Ten simple steps for success; Real weight loss, for real people in the real world, which really works.*

Coming soon:

Do it, Do it, DO IT! *- A Procrastinator's Guide to World Domination*

Stand Up Sexy *- Perfect Posture for Everyday & Better Bedroom Fun. Cure Back Pain - A Doctor's Guide*

Top Ten Finish *- Chasing the coat tails of the ultrarunning elite*

Run a Faster MdS *- A Scientific Guide to Joining the Ultrarunning Elite. Ultramarathon running hints*

references

"If I can see further it is by standing on the shoulders of Giants."
(Isaac Newton, 1676)

Alarcon, G., Eschleman, K., Bowling, N. (2009). Relationships between personality variables and burnout: A meta-analysis. Work & Stress, 23 (3), 244–263.

(Alarcon, Eschleman and Bowling, 2009)

Andrew, L. (2006). Survey Says: Many EPs Suffer in Silence. Emergency Physicians Monthly Online, 13 (3), 1-7.

(Andrew, 2006)

Angela, K., et al. (2012). Embodied Metaphors and Creative "Acts". Psychological Science, 23 (5), 502-509.

(Angela et al, 2012)

Balch, C., et al. (2011). Personal consequences of malpractice lawsuits on American surgeons. Journal of the American College of Surgeons. 213 (5), 657-67.

(Balch et al, 2011)

Baranek, L. (1996). The Effect of Rewards and Motivation on Student Achievement, Masters Theses. Paper 285. Grand Valley

State University. Michigan, US.

(Baranek, 1996)

Beauchamp, T. and Childress, J. (2013). Principles of Biomedical Ethics. 7th ed. USA: Oxford University Press.

(Beauchamp and Childress, 1979)

Belenky, G., et al (2003). Patterns of performance degradation and restoration during sleep restriction and subsequent recovery: a sleep dose-response study. Journal of Sleep Research, 12 (1), 1-12.

(Belenky et al, 2003)

Benassi, V., Sweeney, P., Dufour, C. (1988). Is there a relation between locus of control orientation and depression? Journal of Abnormal Psychology, 97 (3), 357–367.

(Benassi et al, 1988)

Benington, J. and Heller, H. (1995). Restoration of brain energy metabolism as the function of sleep. Progress in Neurobiology, 45 (4), 347-60.

(Benington and Heller, 1995)

Bianchi, R., Schonfeld, I. and Laurent, E. (2015). Is burnout separable from depression in cluster analysis? A longitudinal study. Social Psychiatry and Psychiatric Epidemiology, 50 (6), 1005-11.

(Bianchi et al, 2015)

Brown, D., et al. (2009). Rotating night shift work and the risk of ischemic stroke. American Journal of Epidemiology, 169 (11), 1370-7.

(Brown et al, 2009)

Bourne, T., et al. (2015). The impact of complaints procedures on the welfare, health and clinical practise of 7926 doctors in the UK: a cross-sectional survey. British Medical Journal Open, 5 (1).

(Bourne et al, 2015)

Burn, S. and Oskamp, S. (1986). Increasing Community Recycling with Persuasive Communication and Public Commitment. Journal of Applied Psychology, 16 (1), 29–41.

(Burn and Oskamp, 1986)

Carney, C. and Waters, W. (2006). Effects of a structured problem-solving procedure on pre-sleep cognitive arousal in college students with insomnia. Behavioral Sleep Medicine, 4 (1), 13-28.

(Carney and Waters, 2006)

Charles, S. and Frisch, P. (2005). Adverse Events, Stress, and Litigation: A Physician's Guide. New York: Oxford University Press.

(Charles and Frisch, 2005)

Cialdini, R. (1984). Influence: The Psychology of Persuasion. 1st Collins Business Essentials edition (2007). New York:

Harper Business.

(Cialdini, 1984)

Cole, T. and Carlin, N. (2009). The suffering of physicians. Lancet, 24;374 (9699), 1414-5.

(Cole and Carlin, 2009)

Covey, S. (2004). The 7 Habits of Highly Effective People, Simon and Schuster; New York.

First published in 1989

(Covey, 1989)

Cowan, N. (2001). The magical number 4 in short-term memory: A reconsideration of mental storage capacity. Behavioral and Brain Sciences, 24 (1), 87–114.

(Cowan, 2001)

Creswell, D., et al. (2007). Does Self-Affirmation, Cognitive Processing, or Discovery of Meaning Explain Cancer-Related Health Benefits of Expressive Writing? Personality and Social Psychology Bulletin, 33 (2), 238-250.

(Creswell et al, 2007)

Dale, S. and Olds, J. (2012). Maintaining professionalism in the face of burnout. British Journal of General Practice, 62 (604), 605-607.

(Dale and Olds, 2012)

Danzigera, S., Levavb, J., Avnaim-Pessoa, L. (2011). Extraneous factors in judicial decisions. Proceedings of the National Academy of Sciences, 108 (17), 6889–6892.

(Danzigera et al, 2011)

Dayi - Guangzhou city health department mental health survey.

Baidu.com, (2016). Website. [online] Available at: http://wenku.baidu.com/view/4c906f916bec0975f465e2d2.html (article in Chinese) [Accessed 02 Sep 2016].

(Dayi, 2008)

Demerouti, E., Bakker, A., Nachreiner, F., Schaufeli, W. (2001). The job demands-resources model of burnout. Journal of Applied Psychology, 86 (3), 499–512.

(Demerouti et al, 2001)

The Oldenburg Burnout Inventory: A good alternative to measure burnout and engagement.

Demerouti, E., and Bakker, A. (2008). Handbook of stress and burnout in health care. New York: Nova Science Publishers, pp 65–78.

(Demerouti and Bakker, 2008)

DesRoches, C., Rao, S., Fromson, J., et al. (2010) Physicians' perceptions, preparedness for reporting, and experiences related to impaired and incompetent colleagues. Journal of the American Medical Association, 304, 187-193.

(DesRoches et al, 2010)

Dormann, C., Fay, D., Zapf, D., Frese, M. (2006). A state-trait analysis of job satisfaction: On the effect of core self-evaluations. Applied Psychology: an International Review, 55 (1), 27–51.

(Dormann et al, 2006)

DuPont, R., McLellan, A., Carr, G., Gendel, M., Skipper, G. (2009). How are addicted physicians treated? A national survey of Physician Health Programs. Journal of Substance Abuse Treatment, 37, 1-7.

(DuPont et al, 2009)

Elliott, T., Shewchuk, R., Hagglund, K., Rybarczyk, B., Harkins, S. (1996). Occupational burnout, tolerance for stress, and coping among nurses in rehabilitation units. Rehabilitation Psychology, 41 (4), 267–284.

(Elliott et al, 1996)

Fahrenkopf, A., Sectish, T., Barger, L., et al. (2008). Rates of medication errors among depressed and burnt out residents: prospective cohort study. British Medical Journal, 336 (7642), 488-91.

(Fahrenkopf et al, 2008)

Ferrie, J., et al. (2011). Change in sleep duration and cognitive function: findings from the Whitehall II Study. Sleep, 34 (5), 565-73.

(Ferrie et al, 2011)

Frank, E., Biola, H., Burnett, C. (2000). Mortality rates and causes among U.S. physicians. American Journal of Preventative Medicine, 19 (3), 155-9.

(Frank, Biola and Burnett, 2000)

Frank, E., Dingle, A. (1999). Self-reported depression and suicide attempts among U.S. women physicians. American Journal of Psychiatry, 156 (12), 1887-94.

(Frank and Dingle, 1999)

Frankl, V. (2004). Man's Search for Meaning. New York: Rider.

Originally published in 1946.

(Frankl, 1946)

Freudenberger, H. (1974). Staff burn-out. Journal of Social Issues, 30 (1), 159-165.

(Freudenberger, 1974)

Freudenberger, H., Richelson, G. (1980). Burn Out: The High Cost of High Achievement. What it is and how to survive it. New York: Bantam Books.

(Freudenberger and Richelson, 1980)

Gallicchio, L. and Kalesan, B. (2009). Sleep duration and mortality: a systematic review and meta-analysis. Journal of Sleep Research, 18 (2), 148-58.

(Gallicchio and Kalesan, 2009)

Gawande, A. (2015). Being Mortal: Medicine and What Matters in the End. International: Picador.

(Gawande, 2015)

Goldman, M., Shah, R., Bernstein, C. (2015). Depression and suicide among physician trainees: recommendations for a national response. Journal of the American Medical Association, Psychiatry, 72 (5), 411-2.

(Goldman, Shah and Bernstein, 2015)

Guille, C., Zhao, Z., Krystal, J., Nichols, B., Brady, K., Sen, S. (2015). Web-Based Cognitive Behavioral Therapy Intervention for the Prevention of Suicidal Ideation in Medical Interns: A Randomized Clinical Trial. Journal of the American Medical Association, Psychiatry, 72 (12), 1192-8.

(Guille et al, 2015)

Hätinen, M., Kinnunen, U., Pekkonen, M., Kalimo, R. (2007). Comparing two burnout interventions: Perceived job control mediates decreases in burnout. International Journal of Stress Management, 14 (3).

(Hätinen et al, 2007)

Hawker, L. (2015). Runner: A short story about a long run. New York: Aurum Press Ltd.

(Hawker, 2015)

ICD-10: International Classification of Diseases. (2015). Geneva: World Health Organization.

Ptsd icd 10 - F42.1
Ptsd icd 10 - F43.1

(ICD-10, 2015)

James, W. (1884). What is an Emotion? Mind, 9 (34), 188-205.

(James, 1884)

Jaremko, M., Meichenbaum, D. (2013). Stress Reduction and Prevention.
New York: Springer Science & Business Media.

(Jaremko and Meichenbaum, 2013)

Judge, T., Locke, E., Durham, C. (1997). The dispositional causes of job satisfaction: A core evaluations approach. Research in Organizational Behavior, 19, 151–188.

(Judge, Locke and Durham, 1997)

Judge, T., Erez, A., Bono, J., Thoresen, C. (2002). Are measures of self-esteem, neuroticism, locus of control, and generalized self-efficacy indicators of a common core construct?. Journal of Personality and Social Psychology, 83 (3), 693–710.

(Judge et al, 2002)

Juvenal and Escott. (2015). The Satires Of Juvenal Hardcover. New York: THS, Loeb Classical Library, Andesite Press.

Roman poet Juvenal from his Satires (Satire VI, lines 347–8).

(Juvenal and Escott, 2015)

Kahneman, D. (2012). Thinking, Fast and Slow. London: Penguin.

(Kahneman, 2012)

Kakiashvili, T., Leszek, J., Rutkowski, K. (2013). The medical perspective on burnout. International Journal of Occupational Medicine and Environmental Health, 26 (3), 401-12.

(Kakiashvili, Leszek and Rutkowski, 2013)

Kessler, R., Evelyn, J. (2013). The epidemiology of depression across cultures. Annual Review of Public Health, 34, 119–138.

(Kessler and Bromet, 2013)

Knutson, K., van Cauter, E. (2008). Associations between sleep loss and increased risk of obesity and diabetes. Annals of the New York Academy of Sciences, 1129, 287-304.

(Knutson and van Cauter (2008)

Kraft, U. (2006). Burned Out. Scientific American Mind, June/July 2006, 28-33.

(Kraft, 2006)

Kübler-Ross, E. (1997). Living with Death and Dying: How to communicate with the terminally ill. New York: Scribner.

Originally published in 1969.

(Kübler-Ross, 1969)

Lepper, M., et al. (1973). Undermining children's intrinsic interest with extrinsic reward: A test of the "overjustification" hypothesis. Journal of Personality and Social Psychology, 28 (1), 129-137.

(Lepper et al, 1973)

Luft, J., Ingham, H. (1955). The Johari window, a graphic model of interpersonal awareness. Proceedings of the western training laboratory in group development. Los Angeles University of California, Los Angeles.

(Luft and Ingham, 1955)

Lyubomirsky, S., and Layous, K. (2013). How Do Simple Positive Activities Increase Well-Being? Current Directions in Psychological Science February, 22 (1), 57-62.

(Lyubomirsky and Layous, 2013)

Magdeleine, L. and Schmidt, H. (2011). Self-reflection and academic performance: is there a relationship? Advances in health sciences education : theory and practice, 16 (4), 529–545.

(Magdeleine and Schmidt, 2011)

Maguire, E., Woollett, K., Spiers, H. (2006). London taxi drivers and bus drivers: a structural MRI and neuropsychological analysis. Hippocampus, 16 (12), 1091-101.

(Maguire, Woollett and Spiers, 2006)

Malach-Pines, A., Giora, K. (2005). The Burnout Measure, Short Version. International Journal of Stress Management, 12 (1), 78-88.

(Malach-Pines and Giora, 2005)

Maslach, C., Jackson, S. and Leiter, M. (1996). MBI: The Maslach Burnout Inventory: Manual. Palo Alto: Consulting Psychologists Press.

(Maslach, Jackson and Leiter, 1996)

Maslach, C., Schaufeli, W., Leiter, M. (2001). Job burnout. Annual Review of Psychology, 52, 397–422.

(Maslach, Schaufeli and Leiter, 2001)

Maslow, A. (1943). A theory of human motivation. Psychological Review, 50 (4), 370–96.

(Maslow, 1943)

Mata, D., Ramos, M., Bansal, N., Khan, R., Guille, C., Di Angelantonio, E., et al. (2015). Prevalence of Depression and Depressive Symptoms Among Resident Physicians: A Systematic Review and Meta-analysis. Journal of the American Medical Association, 314 (22), 2373-83.

(Mata et al, 2015)

Mateen, F., Dorji, C. (2009). Health-care worker burnout and the mental health imperative. Lancet, 374 (9690), 595-7.

(Mateen and Dorji, 2009)

McLaurine, W. (2008). A correlational study of job burnout and organizational commitment among correctional officers. Capella University. School of Psychology, pp 92.

(McLaurine, 2008)

Miles, S. (1998). A piece of my mind. A challenge to licensing boards: the stigma of mental illness. Journal of the American Medical Association, 280 (10), 865.

(Miles, 1998)

Miller, G. (1956). The magical number seven, plus or minus two: Some limits on our capacity for processing information. Psychological Review, 63 (2), 81–97.

(Miller, 1956)

Miller, M., Mcgowen, R. (2000). The Painful Truth: Physicians Are Not Invincible. Southern Medical Journal, 93 (10).

(Miller et al, 2000)

Neighbour, R. (2015). The Inner Consultation: How to Develop an Effective and Intuitive Consulting Style, 2nd Ed. London: CRC Press.

First published in 1987.

(Neighbour, 1987)

Neill, M. (2009). You Can Have What You Want. London: Hay

House UK.

(Neill, 2009)

Nevanpera, N., Hopsu, L., Kuosma, E., et al. (2012). Occupational burnout, eating behavior, and weight among working women. American Journal of Clinical Nutrition, 95 (4), 934-43.

(Nevanpera et al, 2012)

---

http://www.nimh.nih.gov/health/statistics/prevalence/major-depression-among-adults.shtml

US National Institute of Mental Health, 2014.

(NIMH, 2014)

Nishi, M., Miyake, H., Kato, T., Yamazoe, M., Tanaka, E., Ishii, T., Usui, K. (1999). Life span of Japanese male medical doctors. Journal of Epidemiology, 9 (5), 315-9.

(Nishi et al, 1999)

Pareto, V. (1896). Cours d'économie politique.

http://www.institutcoppet.org/2012/05/08/cours-deconomie-politique-1896-de-vilfredo-pareto
(free pdf download of both volumes)

(Pareto, 1896)

Park, R., and Searcy, D. (2012). Job Autonomy as a Predictor of Mental Well-Being: The Moderating Role of Quality-Competitive Environment. Journal of Business and Psychology,

27, 305.

(Park and Searcy, 2012)

Kiran, P., Yan, Y., Patel K., Judge, P., Patel, J., Johal, S., Johal, S, Do, P., Leyva, P. (2009). Lifespan and cardiology. British Journal of Cardiology, 16, 299–302.

(Patel et al, 2009)

Pendleton, D., et al. (2003). The New Consultation: Developing Doctor-Patient Communication. Oxford: Oxford University Press.

(Pendelton et al, 2003)

Petersen, M., Burnett, C. (2008). The suicide mortality of working physicians and dentists. Occupational Medicine, 58 (1), 25-9.

(Petersen and Burnett, 2008)

Pinker, S. (1999). How the Mind Works. London: Penguin Press Science.

(Pinker, 1999)

Prochaska, J., Johnson, S. and Lee, P. (1998). The Transtheoretical Model of Behavior Change. In Shumaker, S., Schron, E., Okene, K. and McBee, W. (Eds.) The Handbook of Health Behavior Change 2nd Ed. New York: Springer Publishing Company.

(Prochaska, 1998)

Reis, D., Xanthopoulou, D., Tsaousis, I. (2015). Measuring job and academic burnout with the Oldenburg Burnout Inventory (OLBI): Factorial invariance across samples and countries. Burnout Research,
2 (1), 8–18.

(Reis, Xanthopoulou and Tsaousis, 2015)

Rotter, J. (1966). Generalized expectancies for internal versus external control of reinforcement. Psychological Monographs: General & Applied, 80 (1), 1–28.

Ruotsalainen, J., Verbeek, J., Mariné, A., Serra, C. (2014). Preventing occupational stress in healthcare workers. The Cochrane Database of Systematic Reviews 12: CD002892.

(Ruotsalainen et al, 2014)

Russell, B. (2004). History of Western Philosophy. London: Routledge.

Originally published in 1945.

(Russell, 1945)

Sainte-Beuve, C. (1851). Causeries Du Lundi (Monday Chats). Translated by Trechmann, E. London: Routledge, pp 180.

(Sainte-Beuve, 1851)

Sandstrom, A., Rhodin, L., Olsson, T., Nyberg L. (2005). Impaired cognitive performance in patients with chronic burnout syndrome. Biological Psychology, 69 (3), 271–279.

(Sandstrom et al, 2005)

Sarda. (2016). Reasons by men die earlier that women (sic). Press release. New Delhi: Indian Medical Association (Hqs.). February 23, 2016.

(Sarda, 2016)

Sargent, D., Jensen, V., Petty, T., Raskin, H. (1977). Preventing physician suicide. The role of family, colleagues, and organized medicine. Journal of the American Medical Association, 237 (2), 143-5.

(Sargent et al, 1977)

Scheer, F., et al. (2009). Adverse metabolic and cardiovascular consequences of circadian misalignment. Proceedings of the National Academy of Sciences, 17;106 (11), 4453-8.

(Scheer et al, 2009)

Schernhammer, E., Colditz, G. (2004). Suicide rates among physicians: a quantitative and gender assessment (meta-analysis). American Journal of Psychiatry, 161 (12), 2295-302.

(Schernhammer and Colditz, 2004)

Schwenk, T. (2015). Resident Depression: The Tip of a Graduate Medical Education Iceberg. Journal of the American Medical Association, 314 (22), 2357-8.

(Schwenk, 2015)

Shanafelt, T., Hasan, O., Dyrbye, L., Sinsky, C., Satele, D., Sloan, J., West, C. (2015). Changes in Burnout and Satisfaction With Work-Life Balance in Physicians and the General US Working Population. Between 2011 and 2014. Mayo Clinic Proceedings, 90 (12), 1600-13.

(Shanafelt et al, 2015)

Shirom, A., and Melamed, S. (2005). Does burnout affect physical health? A review of the evidence. In Antoniou, A. Cooper, C. (Eds.) Research companion to organizational health psychology. Cheltenham: Edward Elgar, pp 599-622.

(Shirom and Melamed, 2005)

Spiegel, K., Leproult, R., and van Cauter, E. (1999). Impact of sleep debt on metabolic and endocrine function. Lancet, 23;354 (9188), 1435-9.

(Spiegel, Leproult, and van Cauter 1999)

Spickard, A., Gabbe, S., Christensen, J. (2002). Mid-career burnout in generalist and specialist physicians. Journal of the American Medical Association, 288 (12), 1447-50.

(Spickard, Gabbe and Christensen, 2002)

Starfield, B. (2000). Is US Health Really the Best in the World? Journal of the American Medical Association, 284 (4), 483-485.

(Starfield, 2000)

Stickgold, R., and Matthew, P. (2007). Sleep-Dependent Memory Consolidation and Reconsolidation. Sleep Medicine, 8

(4), 331–343.

(Stickgold and Matthew, 2007)

Thakur, M. (2015). Compassion or empathy? A way forward to reduce GP stress and burnout. British Journal of General Practice, 65 (633), 193.

(Thakur, 2015)

Tversky, A., Kahneman, D. (1974). Judgment under Uncertainty: Heuristics and Biases. Science, 185 (4157), 1124-31.

(Tversky and Kahneman, 1974)

Van Dierendonck, D., Schaufeli, W., Buunk, B. (1998). The evaluation of an individual burnout intervention program: The role of inequity and social support. Journal of Applied Psychology, 83: 392–407.

(van Dierendonck, Schaufeli, and Buunk, 1998)

Van Dierendonck, D., Garssen, B., Visser, A. (2005). Burnout Prevention Through Personal Growth. International Journal of Stress Management, 12 (1), 62-77.

(van Dierendonck et al, 2005)

Voltaire. (1765). Dictionnaire philosophique portatif.

Full download:
https://archive.org/details/dictionnairephi04voltgoog

(Voltaire, 1765)

Walker, M., et al. (2003). Dissociable stages of human memory consolidation and reconsolidation. Nature, 9;425 (6958), 616-20.

(Walker et al, 2003)

West, C., Tan, A., Habermann, T., Sloan, J., Shanafelt, T. (2009). Association of resident fatigue and distress with perceived medical errors. Journal of the American Medical Association, 302 (12), 1294-300.

(West et al, 2009)

Whitelaw, S., Baldwin, S., Bunton, R. and Flynn, D. (2000). The status of evidence and outcomes in Stages of Change research. Health Education Research, 15 (6), 707-718.

(Whitelaw et al, 2000)

Worley, L. (2008). Our fallen peers: a mandate for change. Academy of Psychiatry, 32 (1), 8-12.

(Worley, 2008)

Dr Phil Harley has a lot of letters: MB BS (Lond), MRCGP, DCH, DRCOG, DFFP, DPD, LoC SDI, LoC IUT, PGC MedEd. They aren't important. Mainly this means he is a General Practitioner (primary care physician). He's done medicine for twenty years so far.

He finds the job stressful. This is normal. Probably so do you. This book is about what to do about this and how to recognize, prevent and to treat burnout (which is different from stress) in you, your partner or someone else you know.

www.ingramcontent.com/pod-product-compliance
Lightning Source LLC
Chambersburg PA
CBHW070238190526

45169CB00001B/217